Gabrielle Thompson
9/28/77

S0-BLD-522

MEDICAL EDUCATION IN OKLAHOMA

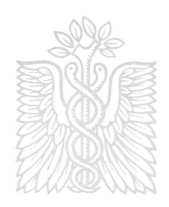

MEDICAL EDUCATION IN OKLAHOMA
The University of Oklahoma School of Medicine and Medical Center 1900–1931

MARK R. EVERETT

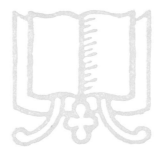

Norman
University of Oklahoma Press

INTERNATIONAL STANDARD BOOK NUMBER: 0–8061–0988–2
LIBRARY OF CONGRESS CATALOG CARD NUMBER: 70–177333

Copyright 1972 by the University of Oklahoma Press, Publishing Division of the University. Composed and printed at Norman, Oklahoma, U.S.A., by the University of Oklahoma Press. First edition.

Preface

MUCH OF THE INFORMATION in this account was not easily attainable and had to be gleaned from a variety of sources. For instance, contemporary officials and faculty members of the University of Oklahoma had no knowledge of the existence or location of the minutes of the first three governing boards of the university. Only after several years of patient and persistent search was I able to examine the records of the Territorial Regents (1893–1906) and of the first State Regents (1908–11), which were found in Evans Hall, in Norman, Oklahoma, through the kindly assistance of Emil R. Kraettli and Mrs. Barbara H. James, of the university regents office. The minutes of the State Board of Education (1911–19) were located at the State Capitol building, in Oklahoma City, as the result of a clue given me by Mel Nash, former Chancellor of the State Regents for Higher Education.

Moreover, files of the office of the dean of the University of Oklahoma School of Medicine prior to 1915 are practically non-existent. This can be understood in view of the fact that earlier deans had their offices at their respective places of private practice.

It is to fill the need for an accessible source of information on the early years of the University of Oklahoma School of Medicine that greater detail has been incorporated into the early chapters of this narrative. I feel greatly rewarded that my long-continued search has made possible the first documented comprehensive history of the University of Oklahoma School of Medicine from 1900 to 1931.[1]

A particular source of gratification to me is that I have been privileged to know personally many of the dedicated and distinguished persons who labored to found and develop medical education in Oklahoma. I have had the advantage of some personal knowledge of each of the deans of the University of Oklahoma School of Medicine following Dean Roy Philson Stoops, with the single exception of Dean Robert F. Williams. I have also known all of the presidents of the university since President Arthur Grant Evans (1908) and all but a few of the teaching physicians who participated in medical education in Oklahoma as early as 1902.

Numerous friends aided me in my search for the early history of the University of Oklahoma School of Medicine. I appreciate and cordially acknowledge their assistance. Former President George L. Cross of the university, Vice-President James L. Dennis and Dean Robert M. Bird of the Medical Center, and the regents of the university made the study possible. Financial assistance came from the School of Medicine and the Medical Sciences Trust Fund. Other officials who furnished considerable information were Emil R. Kraettli, Secretary Emeritus to the regents; M. A. Nash, former Chancellor of the State Regents for Higher Education; Mrs. Barbara James, Secretary to the regents; M. C. Collum, Secretary of the State Board of Education; and Raymond Crews, Business Manager of the Medical Center.

Two senior members of the School of Medicine faculty, Dr. Everett S. Lain and Dr. Wann Langston, both now deceased, gave the author valuable personal background information.

My patient and energetic wife, Alice Allen Everett, and our skilled writer friend, Imogene Patrick, gave excellent editorial advice; Alice revised the manuscript. Karen Kratina and Carolyn Berthelot provided very effective secretarial assistance. Dean Philip E. Smith, Lora Johnson, and Linda Trautman assisted

---

[1] Copies of many of the documents cited have been placed in the library of the School of Medicine.

patiently in making available material in the files of the office of the dean of the School of Medicine.

There were many other friends who gave cheerfully of their time and their knowledge. They include Chancellor E. T. Dunlap of the Oklahoma State Regents for Higher Education; Errett R. Newby, former secretary to the president of the university; Chief Justice Tom Brett of the State Court of Criminal Appeals; Wayne Beal; Mrs. Jennie Dahlgren; Dr. Walter Hartford; Dr. Palmer Howard; Dr. Raymond Murdoch; Dean Helen Patterson of the School of Nursing; and Larry Rember, Secretary to the Alumni Association of the School of Medicine.

Courtesies were extended me when consulting records of the Council on Medical Education and Hospitals in Chicago; the National Archives and National Library of Medicine in Washington; the Oklahoma State Library; the State Historical Library and the Oklahoma County Public Library in Oklahoma City; the main University of Oklahoma Library and Archives at Norman, Professor Arthur McAnally, Director, Professor Arrell M. Gibson, Archivist, and Jack Haley, Assistant Director of Manuscripts Division. Leonard M. Eddy of the Medical Center Library also made every facility available.

The illustrations were gathered from various sources with the help of many individuals and organizations. These sources are shown with the illustrations. I regret that I was unable to obtain photographs of the directors of the School of Nursing for inclusion in this history.

Dean Roy Gittinger's *The University of Oklahoma: 1892–1942* has proved a very dependable source of information. I acknowledge with gratitude the willingness of the University of Oklahoma Press to undertake the publication of this additional contribution to the university's history.

MARK R. EVERETT

Contents

Illustrations

MAP

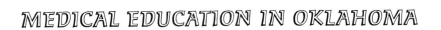

MEDICAL EDUCATION IN OKLAHOMA

Introduction

PROFESSIONAL MOTIVES and national events were powerful
factors from the very beginning in determining the growth of the
University of Oklahoma School of Medicine. To disregard these
contributing elements would result in a sketchy history of this
institution. Therefore, to orient the reader, some brief introductory
information is given in regard to important events and circumstances which helped shape the University of Oklahoma and its
School of Medicine.

The Territory of Oklahoma was established by a congressional
Organic Act in 1890. George W. Steele, of Indiana, was appointed
the first territorial governor. The previous year the Unassigned
Lands, destined to become the initial two million acres of the new
territory, had been opened by Congress to white settlement. The
Unassigned Lands, later called the Oklahoma Lands or Old Oklahoma, lay west of the reservations of the Five Civilized Tribes, in
the very center of the present state. This area comprised the major
portions of the present counties of Canadian, Cleveland, Kingfisher, Logan, Oklahoma, and Payne. It was surrounded by the
Cherokee Outlet, the Sac and Fox country, the Chickasaw Nation,
and the Cheyenne-Arapaho country. The Organic Act of 1890
added to the Territory the distant Panhandle area known as No
Man's Land (old Beaver County). The first federal census in the
region, in 1890, recorded a population of 61,834 in Oklahoma
Territory, with 4,151 in Oklahoma City, 787 in Norman, and
179,321 in the adjoining area of the Five Civilized Tribes.

During the first winter, most of the new towns in the territory instituted tuition common schools, while some rural communities had "subscription" schools. The Organic Act of 1890 provided fifty thousand dollars for temporary support of common schools until the territory could collect property taxes. However, for several years the small fraction of taxable property in the rural areas forced severe limitations on public education, and three-month school terms were prevalent.

The area assigned to the territory continued to increase by extensive additions of lands from the Sac and Fox, Cheyenne-Arapaho, Cherokee, Kickapoo, Kiowa, Comanche, Wichita, Caddo, and Apache reservations, and from Old Greer County, which was transferred from Texas. By 1901, Oklahoma Territory comprised the western half of the present state. Most of the tribes having reservations in the area agreed to the opening of their surplus land for homesteading. This resulted in occupation of vast land areas in a single day.

In 1893, Congress authorized the president to appoint the Dawes Commission to negotiate with the Five Civilized Tribes to abolish tribal titles to their lands, with the express purpose of admitting the Indian Territory to statehood. In 1898, the Curtis Act completely nullified tribal laws and courts and authorized the Dawes Commission to proceed with the allotment of land in severalty, the incorporation of towns, and the establishment of free public schools in the Indian Territory. This action ended the independence of the Five Civilized Nations—the Cherokees, Chickasaws, Choctaws, Creeks, and Seminoles—who had previously come to the Indian Territory from their homes east of the Mississippi River, during the five decades following 1828.

The Curtis Act provided that all tribal governments be terminated on March 4, 1906. By 1907 all tribal lands had been allotted in severalty, the surplus had been opened to white settlement, and Indian reservations no longer existed in Oklahoma.

I. The Territorial University of Oklahoma and Its School of Medicine: 1890–1906

THE UNIVERSITY of Oklahoma was created in 1890 by an act of the First Territorial Legislative Assembly. In June, 1891, the members of the initial Territorial Regents of the University of Oklahoma were appointed by Governor George W. Steele.[1] In July, 1892, David Ross Boyd, of Kansas, became the first president of the university, an office which he continued to hold throughout the territorial period.

The first students enrolled on September 15, 1892. Instruction started in rented quarters on West Main Street, in Norman. None of the 119 students was of college rank, and the courses offered were equivalent to those of the ninth to eleventh grades of high school. Edwin C. DeBarr, Ph.D., a graduate of the University of Michigan, became professor of chemistry and physics in that year, at an annual salary of fifteen hundred dollars. DeBarr was subsequently placed in charge of the pharmacy program organized in 1893 and, in the 1899–1900 yearbook of the university, he was listed as professor of chemistry and pharmacy. In 1900, Professor DeBarr became the senior member of the faculty of the School of Medicine. He remained as professor and head of the Department of Chemistry for thirty-one years and was appointed vice-president of the university in 1909. His university appointments were termi-

---

[1] A list of the members of this board from 1891 to 1907 is in Roy Gittinger, *The University of Oklahoma: 1892–1942* (Norman, University of Oklahoma Press, 1942), 193–95. The first available minutes are those for the regents' meeting of May 6, 1893.

nated on July 1, 1923, in connection with a controversy over the Ku Klux Klan.[2]

By 1898, four years of college courses had been organized. A Department of Biology was established on June 20 of that year. Approximately forty college students were enrolled for the academic year 1898–99, together with three hundred preparatory students. During the same year four students were listed in a newly organized Premedical Department, a division of the College of Arts. This new department included courses in anatomy, chemistry, materia medica, physiology, therapeutics, and toxicology. The specific subjects were taught by the chemistry and biology departments and by the School of Pharmacy. The 1898–99 university catalog indicates that these first premedical students were permitted to choose either a two-year program or a four-year program leading to the degree of Bachelor of Science in the College of Arts. The report of the president of the university to the Territorial Board of Regents for the biennium ending June, 1898, states that "by grouping together appropriate courses from the biological and pharmaceutical departments, and adding others that are required, by a small outlay, a premedical course of two years is offered that will be accepted in medical schools of good standing, as two years of work. There is already a manifest demand for these courses."

The August 1, 1899, minutes of the Territorial Regents record the approval of a motion by Governor Barnes that bona fide citizens of the Five Civilized Indian Tribes be admitted to the university. At the same meeting Albert Heald Van Vleet, who held a Ph.D. from the University of Leipzig, Germany, was appointed professor and head of the new Department of Biology. He supervised the division of premedical studies for one year. According

2 At a special meeting on April 20, 1922, the regents stated that it was unwise for faculty or employees to take an active part in the controversy which then existed in the state over the Ku Klux Klan. At another special meeting on August 15, 1922, a committee of citizens presented a complaint with regard to a commencement address delivered by Professor DeBarr. At a meeting on May 10, 1923, DeBarr was removed from his tenure appointment because the regents felt that he had engaged in political activity and should therefore not retain his position as vice-president of the university.

to the yearbook for the academic year 1899–1900, "The two year course is independent of the College of Arts and is offered to meet the needs of those who desire to devote their entire time to strictly professional studies. Upon completion of the work they will receive a Certificate of Standing. The course aims to cover the first two years of work as given by the best medical schools, and arrangements are being made to have the work accepted by the western medical colleges." Four premedical students were enrolled in 1899–1900.

In 1898, Roy Philson Stoops, later appointed acting dean of the School of Medicine, received one of the first two Bachelor of Arts degrees conferred by the University of Oklahoma in that year. This was the first time the B.A. degree was conferred in either Oklahoma Territory or Indian Territory.

Roy Stoops and Carlton Ross Hume, the other 1898 graduate, became two of the charter members of the first University of Oklahoma Alumni Association, which consisted of the five graduates by 1899. Dr. Stoops, who went on to obtain an M.D. degree, was president of the alumni association in 1904 and 1905. The forty-fifth reunion of the two members of the class of 1898 was held at Dr. Stoops's residence in Oakland, California, in 1943.

Carlton Ross Hume, later Judge Hume, of Anadarko, was the son of Dr. Charles Robinson Hume. A second son, Raymond Robinson Hume, was enrolled in the University of Oklahoma School of Medicine in 1900–1901. He practiced subsequently in Minco, Oklahoma.

Charles Robinson Hume, the father, received his M.D. degree from the University of Michigan in 1874. From 1890 to 1901, he was resident physician in the United States Indian Service on the Kiowa and Comanche Reservation in Anadarko. His presidential address to the Oklahoma State Medical Association at Medicine Park in 1917, reveals the loyalty of this highly respected pioneer physician to the university and its School of Medicine: "A quarter of a century ago, as a pioneer physician in this vicinity, I frequently had occasion to travel the irregular and winding trail blazed between the foothills and mountains of this now famous Wichita

7

range. . . . We have in the Medical Department of the Oklahoma University an institution destined to offer a course equal to that of the sister states. . . . This course from the standpoint of proficiency is equal to that of any one of the twenty-seven state universities that are at present grade A, and heretofore it has only lacked the required hospital facilities. . . . It would seem rational if our lawmakers would exercise a little more solicitude for budding humanity, while doing so much for pigs and calves."[3]

The beginnings of the University of Oklahoma School of Medicine are described by the University of Oklahoma yearbook for 1899–1900:

"With the rapid growth of the Territory and of the University, there is an increasing demand for the establishment of professional departments in the University where students may fit themselves for professional work. The premedical course as outlined aims to prepare the student for advanced standing in accredited medical schools. It will consist of a four years' course and a two years' course. The former may be taken in connection with the regular scientific course and leads to the degree of Bachelor of Science.

"The different lines of work taken up are as follows: general biology, anatomy (human and comparative), histology, physiology, embryology, bacteriology, general chemistry, qualitative chemistry, quantitative chemistry, organic chemistry, physiological chemistry, urinary analysis, toxicology, materia medica, microscopy, pharmacology, pharmaceutical botany.

"NOTE: In 1899–1900 a course in human dissection will be organized. At the last meeting of the Territorial Legislature a bill was passed giving the University the right to use, for purposes of dissection, unclaimed human bodies."[4]

Further information on the beginnings of the School of Medicine is given in a letter from Dr. Roy P. Stoops to Dean Robert U. Patterson, on January 18, 1938.

[3] *Journal of the Oklahoma State Medical Association*, Vol. X (1917), 223.

[4] University of Oklahoma yearbook, 1899–1900, 26. The population of Oklahoma Territory, 61,834 in 1890, had increased to 398,331 by 1900. Oklahoma City had 10,037 residents; Norman, 2,225; Tulsa, 1,390; and Indian Territory, 392,060.

"President Boyd had considerable difficulty in finding a man to head the department [the School of Medicine]. I received a letter from him stating his difficulty and asking me to see what I could do in Chicago. I was only a third year medical student, so I called upon Dr. William A. Evans in Pathology at the University of Illinois. Dr. Evans recommended three physicians. President Boyd corresponded with all three, and finally wrote me that the men would not come for $1,000 a year, and that he had secured the services of Dr. L. N. Upjohn, a graduate of Ann Arbor, Michigan."

Confirmation of this statement is found in an abstract from the minutes of the Territorial Board of Regents for October 2, 1900: "Motion made and seconded that the report of President Boyd be accepted that he had employed Dr. L. N. Upjohn for the Head of the Premedical Department and Director of Physical Culture at a salary of $1,000 per year. Motion made and carried that the estimate [for anatomical supplies] presented by President Boyd and Dr. Upjohn for the Anatomy Department and Premedical Course be approved not to exceed $300 for appropriation."

Two days later the local newspaper, the *Norman Transcript*, commented on the new medical school: "The pharmaceutical course has matured. The course will be fully equal to two years of a full medical course" or the preclinical years as prescribed by the curriculum for a standard school of medicine.[5] A later issue of the *Norman Transcript* went on to say that "the premedical course is almost arranged and will be announced soon. Dr. Upjohn is busy making physical examinations."[6]

Thus, in 1900, seven years before statehood, the first medical school in Oklahoma was officially organized and established at the university in Norman.[7] Dr. Lawrence N. Upjohn served as

---

[5] *Norman Transcript*, October 4, 1900.

[6] *Norman Transcript*, November 28, 1900.

[7] 1900 is the official date of the organization of the University of Oklahoma School of Medicine. However, two prominent national medical publications, the *Journal of the American Medical Association* and the *American Medical Directory*, gave the incorrect date of 1903 in their 1904–1906 and 1906 issues respectively. The University of Oklahoma catalog for 1908–1909 also gave an incorrect date, 1902, notwithstanding the clarifying statement in the 1903–1904 catalog: "In the fall of 1904 the School of

head of the medical course. He was permitted to practice medicine part time during his tenure.[8]

Appointed as instructor in anatomy and physical culture in the biology department, Dr. Upjohn became the third faculty member of this young medical school and the head of its first academic department—anatomy. Tuition was free, and other expenses were estimated at seventy-one and eighty dollars a semester.

Lawrence Northcote Upjohn was born in 1873 into a family of physicians. The founding father, Uriah Upjohn, had migrated from England to the United States in 1832 and received his M.D. degree from the College of Physicians and Surgeons in New York City. Uriah's daughter and three of his sons became physicians. Two of the sons, Dr. Henry U. Upjohn (the father of Lawrence N.) and Dr. William E. Upjohn, entered into a partnership to found the Upjohn Company in Kalamazoo, Michigan. Lawrence Upjohn received his M.D. degree from the University of Michigan in 1900.

In 1904, Dr. L. N. Upjohn resigned as administrator of the University of Oklahoma School of Medicine to join the now-famous drug company founded by his father and uncle, succeeding his uncle as president in 1930 and becoming chairman of the board in 1943. His son, Dr. Everett G. Upjohn, was made president of the Upjohn Company in 1952. Dr. Lawrence N. Upjohn died in 1967, at the age of ninety-three.

Requirements for entrance to the University of Oklahoma in 1900 were as follows: "Those taking the two year course, not candidates for a degree, will be examined before matriculation in the following subjects: English, arithmetic, algebra, physics and Latin. In place of this examination, students may present a

---

Medicine will enter upon its fifth year." It was in 1904 that the University of Oklahoma School of Medicine was first listed in the *Educational Number of the Journal of the American Medical Association*, while the correct organization date (1900) was not recognized in the *Journal* until 1910 or in the *American Medical Directory* until 1934, in its Thirteenth Edition.

8 University of Oklahoma catalog, 1900–1901, Vol. I, No. 1, 40; Eighth Edition of *Polk's Medical Register and Directory of North America*, 1904.

certificate of graduation from high school, normal school or an academy of good standing, or evidence of having passed the entrance examination to a reputable literary or scientific college or university, or a state certificate to teach granted by a state superintendent of public instruction."[9]

Eight students enrolled in the medical course during the academic year 1900–1901. Classes were conducted in the quarters of the biology and chemistry departments and in a small wooden structure (twenty-five by seventy-five feet) which was built for the anatomy courses. Histology and bacteriology were taught by the biology department and chemistry by the chemistry department of the university. The courses in materia medica, pharmacology, and prescription writing were given by the School of Pharmacy. Physiology was presented by the anatomy department.

The course designed to prepare the student for professional work in medicine was called the medical course. "It is intended to add next year to the corps of instructors and to the courses of study. A special circular giving full information concerning work will be issued the first of July."[10] Fees for students were: biology, $1.50; dissection, $10.00, $5.00 for each course; histology, $3.00; bacteriology, $3.00; embryology, $3.00; and chemistry, $17.50. The medical course included the following curriculum.

Freshman Year—First Semester

BIOLOGY: five hours
ANATOMY: course A, human osteology, two hours
            course B, general anatomy, three hours
            course C, practical anatomy, dissections, five hours
GENERAL CHEMISTRY: five hours

Freshman Year—Second Semester

ANATOMY: course D, general anatomy (course B continued),
            four hours

9 University of Oklahoma yearbook, 1899–1900.
10 University of Oklahoma catalog, 1900–1901, Vol. I, No. 1, 41–43.

course E, practical anatomy (course C continued),
five hours

HISTOLOGY: five hours

BACTERIOLOGY: two hours

QUALITATIVE ANALYSIS: five hours

Sophomore Year—First Semester

ORGANIC CHEMISTRY: five hours

QUANTITATIVE ANALYSIS: one hour

MATERIA MEDICA AND PHARMACOLOGY: course A, four hours

PHYSIOLOGY: course A, four hours

EMBRYOLOGY: three hours

ANATOMY OF THE CENTRAL NERVOUS SYSTEM: two hours

Sophomore Year—Second Semester

PHYSIOLOGICAL CHEMISTRY: five hours

MATERIA MEDICA AND PHARMACOLOGY: course B (course A continued),
four hours

PHYSIOLOGY: course B (course A continued), four hours

SURGICAL ANATOMY: three hours

HYGIENE: four hours

It is evident that the University of Oklahoma School of Medicine, at its inception, installed an acceptable curriculum. This accomplishment, only ten years after the Territory of Oklahoma was established, compares very favorably with those of other pioneer territories and states.

The great "land lottery," which opened the lands of the Kiowa-Comanche and Wichita-Caddo reservations to settlement in 1901, expanded Oklahoma Territory into twenty-six counties, the same number existing at statehood. 1901 was also the year in which Oklahoma had three different territorial governors. Early in the year an appropriation bill to finance much-needed buildings for the university was signed by Governor Cassius M. Barnes. Barnes was replaced in May by Governor William M. Jenkins, of Guthrie, who was appointed to the office by President William McKinley, during the first year of his second term as president. Following the

12

assassination of McKinley in September, Vice-President Theodore Roosevelt became president. He removed Governor Jenkins from office, citing official misconduct by the governor in owning stock in the sanitarium at Norman, which held a contract with the territory for the care of patients. Jenkins was replaced by Thompson B. Ferguson of Watonga, owner and editor of the *Watonga Republican*. Ferguson became the seventh territorial governor of Oklahoma, its third governor within a year.

By 1902, the divisions of the university included the College of Arts and Sciences, the School of Pharmacy, the School of Medicine, the School of Fine Arts, and the Preparatory School. In the School of Medicine, which had eight students enrolled in 1901–1902, "two years work consisting of 26 courses or 79 hours is offered. There has been an increased interest in the work of this department. . . . The expansion of the work of the department depends on the finishing of the physiological and anatomical laboratories in the science building. A whole floor, 120 x 60 feet, is given to the work of this department. These laboratories will be equipped and in readiness for the work the latter part of the year."[11]

It appears, however, that only a portion of the floor was finally given to the medical school. The anatomy department was destined to remain in its wooden building until 1924, when construction of a medical school building on the Norman campus was completed. On June 25, 1901, the regents of the university authorized a sum of $200 for the Department of Anatomy for the study of embryology and $325 for physiological apparatus. It appears that there was a tendency to regard this department as the mainstay of the School of Medicine during the early years.[12]

In their 1902 biennial report the regents described the university's medical course: "The School of Medicine was organized to

[11] Biennial Report of the Territorial Board of Regents to Governor Thompson B. Ferguson, June 30, 1902.

[12] The January 28, 1902 minutes of the board of regents refer to the buying of supplies and equipment for the Department of Anatomy as buying them for the "Medical Department."

prepare students for advanced standing in accredited medical schools and to meet the needs of those who desired to devote their entire time to strictly professional studies. The course covers two years of nine months each, and includes the first half of a full four year medical course as given by the best medical colleges, and provides complete and thorough instruction in chemistry, anatomy, physiology, pathology, and pharmacology. These branches form the foundation of medical education, and present conditions demand that at least two years be spent in gaining a working knowledge of them previous to entering upon the study of the more distinctly professional subjects. A number of students have completed the work offered and have entered, with credit, leading medical colleges of the country."

Dr. Upjohn became instructor in anatomy and physiology in 1902 and professor of anatomy and pathology in 1903. Courses in pathology (originally a series of lectures given by a local physician) and also in physics were added to the curriculum in 1902. During the academic year 1902–1903, there were eight students enrolled in the School of Medicine.

In 1903, a number of Oklahoma City physicians met to consider the development of a twenty-thousand-dollar fund for the construction of a medical college building in Oklahoma City, as a clinical facility for the University of Oklahoma School of Medicine. Dr. Archa K. West and Dr. Richard T. Edwards were named as a committee of two to contact physicians regarding the proposal.[13] This activity was doubtless related to a later conference:

"In 1903, Dr. H. Coulter Todd was asked by a group of Oklahoma City physicians to arrange a conference with the authorities of the Territorial University at Norman, and President Boyd selected Dr. Upjohn to represent the University at the conference. Others present were Drs. A. K. West, Lea A. Riely, L. Haynes Buxton and H. Coulter Todd. Dr. Upjohn reported unfavorably on their proposal to found a medical school including the clinical subjects. President Boyd subsequently informed the physicians

13 *Daily Oklahoman*, April 22, 1903.

14

that the establishment of a four year college of medicine within the Territorial University would be postponed indefinitely."[14]

In 1903, Roy Philson Stoops, M.D., later destined to become head of the School of Medicine, was appointed instructor in physiology, at an annual salary of five-hundred dollars, and David Connolly Hall, M.S., was designated instructor in pharmacology, making a total of five faculty members for the medical school. The enrollment of only five students for the year 1903–1904, indicates that applications for entrance into the School of Medicine were languishing.

In the fall of 1904, the University of Oklahoma School of Medicine entered on its fifth session. According to the university catalog for that year, "no clinical courses are offered, and it is deemed best that hospital and clinical instruction should be deferred until a student enters upon his third year. Those who have finished in a satisfactory manner the two year course given by this university are admitted to advanced standing in other medical schools, and will be able to graduate in medicine after two more years of study."

In 1904, Dr. L. N. Upjohn resigned his position at the university. Dr. Roy Philson Stoops succeeded him as director of the medical department and instructor in anatomy.

Dr. Stoops was born in Winona, Minnesota, in 1877. He received his M.D. degree from the University of Illinois in 1903. In the same year he married Eunice Gertrude Rand, M.D., a graduate of the American Medical Missionary College. Various issues of the *Norman Transcript* between November 3, 1904, and May 11, 1905, carried his professional announcement: "Dr. R. P. Stoops, M.D., Physician and Surgeon, and Eunice R. Stoops, M.D., Diseases of Women and Children, have their private office in the back of the First National Bank Building in Norman."

A word of explanation may be helpful in understanding the peculiar administrative titles used in connection with the School

[14] Gaston Litton, *History of Oklahoma* (New York, Lewis Historical Publishing Co., 1957), II, 376, 403, 404. See also H. Coulter Todd, "History of Medical Education in Oklahoma, 1904–1910," *Bulletin of the University of Oklahoma, University Studies,* No. 26 (1928), 27.

15

of Medicine from its inception in 1900 to 1907. Dr. Upjohn was originally appointed as head of the premedical course in 1900, which was occasionally referred to as the medical course during the period 1900–1903, and as the School of Medicine in 1903–1904. When Dr. Stoops became the administrator in 1904, he continued with the designation head or director, until 1907, when his title was changed to that of acting dean. Apparently David R. Boyd, president of the university, opposed delegating executive authority and having any deans preside over autonomous colleges. However, it became necessary to use an acceptable title after the School of Medicine became a member of the Association of American Medical Colleges in 1906. The term, acting dean, was then employed.[15]

During the period 1904–1905, James Seymour, Ph.C., as instructor in pharmacy, and Frank E. Knowles, Ph.B., as instructor in physics, were added to the faculty of the School of Medicine, making a total of six members. Seven students were enrolled in the school.[16] In 1905, students in the School of Medicine and the School of Pharmacy organized the Society of Pharmo-Medics, which lasted only two years. Construction of the new Science Hall was still in progress in the spring of 1904, and the building was finally occupied later in the year.

The December 8, 1904, minutes of the regents reported that the estimated expense for the entire university for the upcoming biennium would be $62,325 a year. The *Session Laws of Oklahoma Territory* indicate that a levy of $50,000 a year was authorized for the benefit of the university in 1905, in addition to approximately $9,000 from land leases.

According to the March, 1906, catalog there were sixteen students in the school during 1905–1906. The faculty of nine consisted of Roy Philson Stoops, M.D., instructor in anatomy and

---

[15] Roy P. Stoops to Robert U. Patterson, January 18, 1938.

[16] The *Educational Numbers of the Journal of the American Medical Association* give annual information concerning the numbers of faculty members and of students enrolled. At times these figures do not agree with those of the university catalog. The author has chosen the catalogs as the most direct and correct source of this information.

director of the school; Edwin DeBarr, Ph.D., professor of chemistry; Cyril Methodius Jansky, B.S., professor of physics and electrical engineering; Albert Heald Van Vleet, Ph.D., professor of biology; Homer Charles Washburn, Ph.C., B.S., professor of pharmacy and materia medica; Charles Sharp Bobo, M.D., lecturer on forensic medicine; Joseph Melville Finney, M.D., Assistant in osteology and model maker; David Connolly Hall, M.S., instructor in pharmacology; and Edward Marsh Williams, A.B., B.S., instructor in pathology and histology.[17]

The minutes of the April 19, 1905, meeting of the regents indicate that few salaries had been improved. For instance, Professor DeBarr, professor of chemistry, received $1,800 a year; Dr. R. P. Stoops, director of the School of Medicine and instructor in anatomy, received $600 for the year 1905–1906, and Dr. Finney, M.D., assistant in osteology and model maker, received $1,000.

Dr. Finney, a native of Oklahoma, was immediately engaged for work at the university after he showed President Boyd a statue he had carved. His appointment as model maker was first reported in the 1904–1905 university catalog. The 1908–1909 catalog indicates that Dr. Finney was still the university model maker in 1907–1908, and that the Biology Museum preserved his models of animals and dissections. *The American Medical Directory* reports that Dr. Finney practiced in Oklahoma City from 1909 to 1921. He was on the faculty of the Epworth College of Medicine as junior professor of anatomy from 1908 to 1910, and in 1912 was professor of surgery and anatomy in the Southwest Postgraduate Medical College. Both schools were located in Oklahoma City. In 1921, he resided at the Masonic Home near El Reno, Oklahoma. He died in 1922 at age fifty-three.

According to a university publication in 1906: "During the past few years the courses of the medical colleges have been in great part revised so that the fundamental studies in general subjects are taken before special courses and advanced work may

[17]Edward Marsh Williams was originally appointed by the regents as instructor of histology and embryology.

17

be pursued. As outlined below, it will be seen that our work includes these fundamental and general subjects so arranged that a student on completing them, may enter any of the better medical colleges and continue his work without break or confusion in his course, and receive his degree in two more years."

Further information followed a detailed outline of the courses: "General equipment includes the laboratories and equipment of Science Hall and the Anatomical Building. On the first floor of Science Hall are the laboratories of chemistry and pharmacy, with rooms for work in general chemistry, organic chemistry and physiological chemistry, qualitative and quantitative chemical analysis, pharmacy and pharmacognosy. On the second floor are the biological laboratories with rooms for normal and pathological histology, bacteriology, embryology, physiology and pharmacology.

"The anatomical building contains a large dissecting room, many anatomical charts and models and the departmental library. The departmental collections of books in the laboratories are intended for daily reference and are at all times accessible.

"The necessary expense of living need not exceed $3.50 to $4.00 per week. Prospective students are advised not to buy second-hand copies of medical books as the introduction of a new terminology in anatomy and other subjects renders many such difficult or impossible to use in classwork."[18]

Fees for students were: biology and embryology, $3.00; dissection, $15.00; histology, $3.00; bacteriology, $3.00; embryology, $3.00; pathological histology, $6.00; and physiology, $3.00. In addition there were required deposits: general chemistry, $5.00; qualitative analysis, $5.00; physiological chemistry, $10.00; quantitative analysis, $2.50; and osteology, $5.00.

Courses for the first year included dissection, embryology, general biology, general chemistry, histology, osteology, physics, physiology, and qualitative analysis; for the second year, bacteriology, general pathology, neurology, organic chemistry, patho-

18 *Sixth Annual Session, 1905–1906, School of Medicine*, Norman, University of Oklahoma, 1906.

logical histology, pharmacognosy, pharmacology, physiological chemistry, physiology, and surgical anatomy.

In 1906 the University of Oklahoma School of Medicine was accepted into membership in the Association of American Medical Colleges.[19] This achievement, one year before statehood, was confirmed by President Evans of the university and by Dr. Stoops, who, in his letter to Dean Robert U. Patterson, recalled that it was during his administration that this event had occurred, and that it was indeed through his effort that acceptance into membership had transpired.[20] The 1907 report by the Territorial Board of Regents of the University of Oklahoma to the Honorable Charles N. Haskell, first governor of the State of Oklahoma, also announced that "the School of Medicine was admitted to membership in the Association of American Medical Colleges on March 19, 1906, after a rigid examination by its representative, Dr. Henry B. Ward."[21] Two years later, Dr. Ward, dean of the medical department at the University of Nebraska, was elected president of the Association of American Medical Colleges.[22]

From that day to this, the University of Oklahoma School of Medicine has remained a member of the association. It has been the only medical school from Oklahoma admitted to the association despite the claims of certain other schools.

The 1907 report of the Territorial Board of Regents also noted that: "As now constituted, the School of Medicine embraces the following departments of instruction which were organized as such in 1906: *Anatomy*, instruction is offered in the following subdivisions: dissection, osteology, histology and neurology. Material for dissection is abundant and is procured according to

[19] *Journal of the American Medical Association*, Vol. XLVII (1906), 633.

[20] *Sooner Magazine* (August 7, 1939), 27. Dean Patterson stated incorrectly that it was in 1901.

[21] Payment of expenses of Dr. Henry B. Ward's visit was authorized at the March 3, 1906 regents' meeting. The last available minutes of the board are those for the April 27, 1906 meeting.

[22] *University Umpire*, Vol. IX, No. XII (April 1, 1906), 15–16; *University Umpire*, Vol. IX (May 15, 1906), 20–21. These two issues contain interesting details concerning the School of Medicine for 1905–1906.

the provision of the Session Laws of 1899. *Chemistry*, instruction is offered in the following subdivisions: general chemistry, analytical chemistry, quantitative chemistry, organic chemistry and physical chemistry. *Forensic Medicine*, instruction given one hour per week throughout the year. *Pathology*, subdivisions: general bacteriology, bacteriological analysis, research bacteriology, parasitology, general pathology and special pathology. *Physiology*, subdivisions: human physiology, experimental animal physiology, pharmacology and materia medica. The subjects of pathology and bacteriology were organized in 1906 as a division of the Botany Department."[23] The course in physics was discontinued at the close of the 1905–1906 academic year.

There were ten faculty members in the School of Medicine during the year 1906–1907; new appointments in 1906 included Henry Higgins Lane, M.A., professor of zoology and embryology, and William Gladstone Lemmon, B.S., assistant in pathology and bacteriology. Edward M. Williams, upon becoming instructor in pathology and bacteriology in 1906, was temporarily in charge of the department.[24] Williams was dropped from the faculty in 1908, together with President Boyd and Acting Dean Roy Stoops. Dr. Stoops, who was appointed instructor in physiology and bacteriology in 1903, and director of the medical department and instructor in anatomy in 1904, became professor of anatomy in 1906, thus becoming head of that department.[25] Dr. Charles Sharp Bobo was now the head of the Department of Forensic Medicine.

There were thirteen students enrolled in the School of Medicine in 1906–1907.

23 In his article in the *Sooner Magazine* (August, 1939), 27, Dean Robert U. Patterson stated erroneously that the physiology department was organized in 1908.

24 Notes in possession of Louis Alvin Turley, December 5, 1938.

25 Gittinger, *The University of Oklahoma*, 196, 45.

II. Professional Influence on Medical Education

THE DEVELOPMENT of medical schools throughout our nation, and in Oklahoma as well, resulted largely from certain nonacademic forces which exerted powerful influences. Among these were the actions of professional medical societies, which led to the incorporation of schools of medicine into the universities; the medical practice acts and licensing examinations of the individual states, which supplanted the old apprenticeship system; the expanding application of science to medicine; and economic support by the state governments and more recently by the federal government.

It should be noted that both medical examinations and licensing developed in parallel fashion with medical education and that the American Medical Association originated in connection with efforts of physicians to raise the standards of medical education and licensing.

The several local medical associations, whose leaders played direct roles in the development of medical education in Oklahoma, merit special mention.

The Indian Territory Medical Association was formed at Muskogee as early as April 18, 1881, with Dr. B. F. Fortner, of Claremore, as its first president. Two subsequent officials, Dr. Francis B. Fite of Muskogee, president 1893–94, and Dr. LeRoy Long of Caddo, president 1900–1901, were very influential in the development of the four-year School of Medicine of the University of Oklahoma.

21

The Oklahoma Territorial Medical Association was established on May 9, 1893, with Dr. Delos Walker of Oklahoma City as its first president. Subsequent presidents who became active clinical professors in the School of Medicine were Dr. John A. Hatchett of El Reno, president 1897–98; Dr. Abraham L. Blesh of Guthrie, president 1903–1904; and Dr. Archa K. West of Oklahoma City, president 1904–1905.

At a joint convention of the two territorial medical societies on May 7–9, 1906, the Oklahoma State Medical Association was founded, with Dr. B. F. Fortner, now from Vinita, as its first president. At this meeting Dr. West, dean of the Epworth College of Medicine, Oklahoma City, gave an address on medical education.[1] Members of the faculty of the University of Oklahoma who became presidents of the association prior to 1964 were Dean Charles S. Bobo, 1907–1908; Dr. John W. Riley, 1914–15; Dean Lewis J. Moorman, 1919–20; Dr. John W. Duke, 1920; Dr. Everett S. Lain, 1924–25; Dr. Edmund S. Ferguson, 1929–31; Dean LeRoy Long, 1934–35; Dr. Henry H. Turner, 1940–41; Dr. Charles R. Rountree, 1944–45; Dr. George H. Garrison, 1949–50; Dr. L. Chester McHenry, 1951–52; Dr. Rufus Q. Goodwin, 1955–56; and Dr. John F. Burton, 1957–58.

In 1901 the American Medical Association was thoroughly reorganized, converting it into an effective representative body for the whole country and the entire medical profession. In the following year, 1902, the association appointed a committee on medical education to study the national situation and to bring in a report.

That committee recommended in 1904 the creation of a Council on Medical Education, to be appointed by the president of the American Medical Association, and the employment of a permanent secretary for the council. Through the action of the house of delegates of the association, it was decided that appointment of all members of the council must be confirmed by the house of delegates. The functions of the council, as stated at that time, were to make an annual report on the existing conditions of medical education in the United States, to make suggestions as to the means

1 *Oklahoma Medical News-Journal*, Vol. XIV (1906), 145.

and methods by which the American Medical Association might best influence medical education favorably, and to act as the agent of the American Medical Association in its efforts to elevate medical education.

The Council on Medical Education was destined to become the national guardian of educational requirements for physicians and an anathema to those who trifled with that objective. The council was of extreme importance in the development of the world's most effective system of medical education.

At this point it is important to review the interrelations of the Association of American Medical Colleges and the Council on Medical Education in the accreditation of medical colleges.

A national organization known as the American Medical College Association existed from 1876 to 1882, during which time Dr. Leartus Connor was its secretary. In 1882, due to the loss of a number of the founding member colleges, the association and its efforts to raise the standards of medical education came to an end. However, in 1890 the present organization, known as the Association of American Medical Colleges, was formed. Dr. Fred Z. Zapffe became secretary-treasurer of this association in 1903, a post which he held until 1948. One of his first official duties was to visit and survey each member school. Six of these schools were still being rated as class B schools by the Council on Medical Education ten years later. By 1918 there were fifty-six member colleges in class A and three in class B.

Surveys of the medical schools became the joint endeavor of the Council on Medical Education and the Association of American Medical Colleges in 1919, at which time there were eighty-five medical schools. A Liaison Committee on Medical Education was formed in 1942, with equal membership from the two organizations. It conducted the surveys following that date. As stated by Dr. Dean F. Smiley, who was appointed secretary of the Association of American Medical Colleges in 1948, "This arrangement guarded against 'guild control' of the profession and 'ivory tower control' of medical educators." In 1952 a requirement of three years of preliminary college work for admission of students into its member schools was initiated by the association. Five years later Dr. Ward Darley became executive director of the Association of American Medical Colleges.[2]

A partial summary of the activities of the Council on Medical Education follows: The American Medical Association appointed a committee, with Dr. Arthur D. Bevan as chairman, to survey the status of medical education in 1902. In 1905, Dr. N. P. Colwell became the first secretary of the Council on Medical Education. At the annual conference that year, a four-year high school diploma and a four-year medical course following it were advocated for medical students. Dr. Bevan stated that by 1905, when the council held its first conference on medical education, very few of the American medical schools had made any noteworthy improvement during the previous twenty years. Only five schools required two or more years of preliminary training in the university prior to entrance into medical school.[3]

In 1906 there were more than one hundred and sixty medical colleges in the United States, too many of which were mere diploma mills. Dr. Bevan stated: "I remember as well as though it were yesterday, although it was twenty two years ago, that . . . I said, 'it is evident from a study of the medical schools of this country, and their work, that there are five especially rotten spots which are responsible for most of the bad medical instruction. They are Illinois with fifteen medical schools, Missouri with fourteen medical schools, Maryland with eight medical schools, Kentucky with seven medical schools, and Tennessee with ten medical schools. That is, fifty four medical schools in these five states, and not more than six of these can be considered acceptable!'

"These startling figures led to an immediate and drastic reform. As the council continued to study the problem, it soon became

2 The information concerning the Association of American Medical Colleges was obtained largely from Dean F. Smiley, "History of the Association of American Medical Colleges," *Journal of Medical Education*, Vol. XXXII (1957), 512–25.

3 Arthur D. Bevan, "Cooperation in Medical Education and Medical Service, Functions of the Medical Profession of the University, and of the Public," *Journal of the American Medical Association*, Vol. XC (1928), 1173.

24

evident that the most important piece of work to be done by the council was to make a personal inspection by the board of the 160 schools. The country was divided into sections, and each of the 160 or more schools was visited by some member of the council or by the secretary, Dr. Colwell, in most instances by the secretary and some member of the council."[4] According to the records of the Council on Medical Education, Dr. Colwell visited every medical school during the period 1906–1907.

4 *Ibid.*, 1174.

III. Medical Education in the State of Oklahoma: 1907–1909

BY 1905, with the work of the Dawes Commission completed and the tribal governments and common ownership of land terminated, the Indian Territory was in a position to petition for statehood. So it was that the year 1907 marked the end of the "Twin Territories"—Indian Territory and Oklahoma Territory—as political subdivisions of the United States. Consequently, this was the last year of the Territorial Board of Regents, which was terminated on December 21, 1907.

Between 1890–1907, a period in which executive and judicial officers of Oklahoma Territory were appointed by the president, there had been eight governors: George W. Steele, 1890–91; Robert Martin, 1891–92; Abraham J. Seay, 1892–93; William C. Renfrow, 1893–97; Cassius M. Barnes, 1897–1901; William M. Jenkins, 1901; Thompson B. Ferguson, 1901–1906; and Frank Frantz, 1906–1907. Of this number, only Governor Renfrow was a Democrat; the others were Republicans.

Despite a petition for the admission of Indian Territory into the Union as the proposed State of Sequoyah, with a constitution approved by the voters in Indian Territory, the United States Congress accepted the constitution for the proposed State of Oklahoma. An enabling act (signed June 16, 1906) joined Oklahoma Territory and Indian Territory, thus forming the single state of Oklahoma.

On November 20, 1906, the Oklahoma Constitutional Convention met in Guthrie, with Henry S. Johnston of Perry as the

Democratic caucus chairman. William H. Murray, known as the "Sage of Tishomingo," was elected president of the convention, and Charles N. Haskell was elected the majority leader.[1] The state constitution which evolved followed the Enabling Act of 1906 in detail and was approved by the voters on September 17, 1907. Although President Roosevelt was not exactly pleased with the 1906 act, he acted with expediency and issued a proclamation on November 16 announcing the admission of Oklahoma to the Union.

There was a total population of 1,414,177 in the new state at the time of admission—more than in some of the other states of the Union and about four times as many as in any other state when admitted into the Union. Oklahoma was then the leading oil-producing state. Oklahoma City's population had grown to 32,452 and that of Tulsa to 7,298.

Many progressive Oklahomans had become impatient with the federal appointees and "Republican obstructionism" of territorial days, and many people in both territories were discontented with their carpetbag territorial authorities. David Ross Boyd was serving in his sixteenth year as president of the university. Rumors were widespread that considerable reorganization, not only of the university faculty but of the university itself, might be expected under the new state government.

At the primary election in June, 1907, made mandatory by the constitutional convention of November, 1906, Charles N. Haskell won the Democratic nomination for governor, defeating Lee Cruce of Ardmore. Haskell went on to become the first governor of Oklahoma, serving from 1907 to 1911. In the first legislature (December, 1907–March, 1909) Henry S. Johnston of Perry was president pro tempore of the senate, and William H. Murray was

---

1 Robert L. Williams, another delegate, was a Democratic national committeeman from Indian Territory at the time and a potential candidate for governor of the new state. He and Murray were political rivals, sharing a mutual distrust of one another, but Haskell was able to bring the two antagonists together. The three formed a powerful triumvirate which was to have great meaning for the development of the University of Oklahoma School of Medicine. One of the three was destined to appear as a most effective friend of the School of Medicine, while another would become a carping meddler in university affairs.

27

the speaker of the house. Robert L. Williams was selected as chief justice of the state supreme court.

Oklahoma fortunately had as its first governor a person of great ability and wide experience in business and government. Governor Haskell was very popular from the start. He ruled with an iron hand and proved to be one of the most capable public officials that Oklahoma has had. He was an ex officio member of the new Board of Regents of the University of Oklahoma, which was composed entirely of new members.[2] The first president of the board was Lee Cruce of Ardmore, who resigned in 1910 and became the second governor of Oklahoma in 1911, the same year in which the state regents, as governing board of the university, was replaced by the state board of education.

In 1907 the Council on Medical Education initiated its first classification of medical schools. Class A indicated that the school was approved and acceptable, class B corresponded to the modern classification of "on probation," and class C was unacceptable. Classification was based on the following factors: the showing of graduates before state examining boards; the requirements for preliminary education; the character of the medical curriculum; the medical school's plan, instruction, laboratory facilities, dispensary facilities, hospital facilities, libraries, museums, charts, and teaching equipment; the extent to which teachers in the first two years devoted their entire time to teaching and showed evidence of research; and the extent to which the school was conducted for profit rather than teaching. Of the 160 schools classified, there were 82 in class A, 46 in class B, and 32 in class C.

The University of Oklahoma School of Medicine, which had been inspected in the spring of 1907[3] by Dr. N. P. Colwell, representing the Council on Medical Education, was rated as in class A. There were seven medical schools offering no more than

---

2 A list of the members of the board from 1907 to 1911 is given in Gittinger, *The University of Oklahoma*, 199. The first available record of a meeting of these regents is from August 7, 1908, although the act creating the board was approved December 21, 1907.

3 Erroneously stated as 1909 by Robert U. Patterson in his article "Medical School has 964 Graduates," *Sooner Magazine*, Vol. XI (August 7, 1939), 27.

the first two years of medical education, including the University of Oklahoma and the University of Wisconsin.

It was in 1907 that Dr. Roy Philson Stoops was appointed acting dean of the school and Guy Yandell Williams, B.A., instructor in chemistry joined the medical faculty. During the year E. Marsh Williams was temporarily in charge of the Department of Pathology.

For the year 1907–1908, the university recorded an enrollment of fifteen students in the School of Medicine; included in the list were two future members of the medical faculty, Rex Bolend and Roscoe Walker.

The report of the Territorial Board of Regents to Governor Charles N. Haskell, for June, 1905–June, 1907, contained a pertinent summary: "This department [the medical course] was organized in 1900 to enable graduates in the College of Arts and Sciences to obtain advanced standing in medical colleges and for the benefit of students who desired to devote their entire time to professional studies while attending the university. After completing either course, the student can obtain admission to the junior class in most leading medical colleges in the United States. The following institutions have expressed themselves as willing to give full credit: University of Nebraska, University of Illinois, St. Louis University, Washington University at St. Louis, Jefferson Medical College, Cornell University, and under certain conditions, Harvard University, Chicago University and Western Reserve University.

"The School of Medicine maintains high standards in regard to preliminary education required of each applicant for matriculation. But in this regard the law regarding the licensing of medical practitioners is lamentably deficient. Legislation is needed requiring that all applicants for license to practice medicine submit evidence of having had four years of high school work, and after January, 1910, an additional year of college work in physics, chemistry, biology and language. This policy is supported by both the Council on Medical Education and the Association of American Medical Colleges, and many of the states have already enacted laws requiring this amount of general education. Two states, Kentucky and Minnesota, are even more stringent in their requirements. The students who have completed work in medicine here have all entered medical colleges and in every case have acquitted themselves with credit."

Within the final eight years of the period of territorial status for Oklahoma, under the guidance of President David Ross Boyd, the University of Oklahoma School of Medicine had been established, a satisfactory curriculum had been developed, and the medical faculty had increased from three to ten members. That the enrollment response was disappointingly low was due largely to the generally unsatisfactory status of medical education throughout the nation. Inspections and surveys leading to the *Flexner Report*, which signaled the end of a number of schools of medicine, were under way at the close of this period. Only half of the medical schools achieved an acceptable class A rating. Much credit is due the two youngest deans in the entire history of the University of Oklahoma School of Medicine. Well-trained and capable physicians, each aged twenty-seven at the time of his appointment, they both served effectively under conditions of austerity to make the School of Medicine one of the class A schools in 1907.

The June, 1909, catalog of the University of Oklahoma lists ten members of the faculty of the School of Medicine for the year 1908–1909. John Dice Maclaren, M.S., M.D., became professor of physiology and therapeutics, head of the Department of Physiology, and secretary of the faculty in 1908. Walter Leander Capshaw, M.D., was appointed professor of anatomy to replace Dr. Stoops, and Louis Alvin Turley, M.A., became instructor in pathology and neurology and also bacteriologist for the state board of health. Dr. Turley had obtained his degree in pathology from Harvard University; in 1916 he received a Ph.D. from the same institution. His appointment as instructor was recorded in the June, 1908, catalog, but on August 7, he was promoted to professor of pathology and neurology and became head of the Department of Pathology and Bacteriology. At the same time,

Robert Hickman Riley was appointed a laboratory assistant in that department.

In 1908, Governor Haskell named Dr. J. C. Mahr the state commissioner of health. The state health department offices were located at Guthrie, but the laboratory division was at the University of Oklahoma, under the direction of Professor Edwin DeBarr.

The Session Laws for 1908 show yearly state appropriations of $91,081 for the support and maintenance of the university during the 1908–1910 biennium.

The report of the board of regents to Governor Charles N. Haskell, for 1907 to October, 1908, states: "We are able to insure students that they will be received into any of the medical schools of the Association of American Medical Colleges so as to carry on their work from the point to which we take them here. We must, however, look forward to the time before long when the state of Oklahoma shall offer its own people the opportunity for a complete and thorough medical training."

Charles F. Long stated in his history of the University of Oklahoma that the "actuality of statehood, followed by the election of Charles N. Haskell as the State's first governor, resulted in an almost complete upheaval of the University faculty. President Boyd was classed as an aristocrat, not democratic enough, by Governor Haskell, and was summarily discharged of his duties. . . . [Later] President Brooks stated, 'Although Dr. Boyd had things worked out fine until his discharge, the school had gone to pot when he left. Everywhere there were signs of political interference. The Democrats had tried their best to root out all evidences of the preceding Republican territorial administration. . . .'

"[President] Joseph H. Brandt also analyzed it succinctly. . . . 'His [Boyd's] republicanism wasn't palatable to the staunch new democracy! Asked to leave also were several others, and with the firings came hirings, both from a totally new Board of Regents appointed by the new Governor.' "[4]

The subject of political interference in the state university was

4 Charles F. Long, "With Optimism for the Morrow, a History of the University of Oklahoma," *Sooner Magazine*, Vol. XXXVIII (September, 1965), 26, 34, 35.

discussed in at least one newspaper. "Shall the People Rule in Oklahoma? . . . Last March, under a ruling of the Attorney General, the control of the State University was taken from the Board of Regents and vested in the Board of Education. Immediately thereafter, Dr. Boyd was removed from the presidency of the university, and Mr. A. Grant Evans, who had done effective campaign work for the Governor, was appointed in his place. The Supreme Court of the State reversed the ruling of the Attorney General, and so undid the work of the Board of Education. The Board of Regents of the State University thereupon proceeded to reverse its former action and even outdo the action of the Board of Education. President Boyd was a second time removed, and with him more than a third of the faculty, including three out of four deans, four heads of departments, an assistant professor, the treasurer, and several instructors. . . . The removal could not be an endeavor to secure superior scholarship. . . . The removal could not be due to the 'pernicious activity' in politics of the persons removed. None of them were active in politics. President Boyd, although a Republican, never belonged to any political organization, never attended a political convention in the state, even as a spectator, and never inquired into, and never knew, unless by accident, the political views of any member of the faculty."[5] After leaving the University of Oklahoma, Boyd served as president of the University of New Mexico from 1912 to 1919.

Rev. Arthur Grant Evans,[6] elected president of the university on June 23, 1908, took office on July 1. The June date refers to the

[5] Unindexed papers in the possession of Stratton Brooks; editorial by Lyman Abbott from *The Outlook*, reprinted in the *Oklahoma City Times*, September 5, 1908. The principal charge against President Boyd was that he had engaged in politics. A friendly suit filed with the state supreme court in early April was said to have been brought at the request of Governor Haskell, President Lee Cruce of the board of regents, and State Superintendent of Public Instruction E. D. Cameron.

[6] Arthur Grant Evans was born in India. He came to the Indian Territory years before he became a colleague of Governor Haskell and his faithful ally as a delegate to the Sequoyah separatist statehood convention. He was president of Henry Kendall College, a Presbyterian school which had previously been moved from Muskogee to Tulsa and was the antecedent of the University of Tulsa. An editorial in the June 20, 1908 issue of the *Oklahoma City Times* portrayed Rev. Evans as an upright Christian gentleman.

action of the newly appointed state board of regents. Prior to this the State Board of Education met on March 20, 1908. The minutes of this meeting state that "Governor Haskell placed A. Grant Evans of Tulsa in nomination for the position of President of the University of Oklahoma. Mr. Evans was unanimously elected, his term of office to commence on July 1, 1908." Present were Governor C. N. Haskell, State Superintendent of Public Instruction E. D. Cameron, Attorney General Charles West, and Secretary of State William M. Cross.

In the summer of 1908, Dean Stoops, Professor Cyril Jansky, and Edward M. Williams were dropped from the faculty concurrently with the dismissal of President Boyd.[7] Dr. Stoops continued to practice medicine in Norman for a while and later practiced in Amarillo and Crosbyton, Texas, and in Mitchell and Scottsbluff, Nebraska. Also, for a time, he was a captain in the medical corps and chief of the otolaryngology service at Base Hospital, Camp Pike, Arkansas. In 1925, he commenced practice in Oakland, California. Dr. Stoops was listed in the 1950 *American Medical Directory* as conducting an ear, eye, nose, and throat practice in Oakland. He died that same year.

Dr. Charles Sharp Bobo became dean of the School of Medicine and professor of forensic medicine on September 1, 1908. He remained in that position until September 1, 1911. His tenure covered the time when the University of Oklahoma School of Medicine changed from a two-year to a four-year school.

Dr. Bobo was born in 1856. He received his M.D. degree from the Louisville Medical College in 1881 and came to Norman in 1898. Dr. Bobo, a pleasant and popular general practitioner, was president of the Oklahoma State Medical Association in 1907–1908. He remained a practicing physician and surgeon in Norman until 1940. He died in 1942.

The university quarterly bulletin for the School of Medicine for

---

[7] In the minutes of the April 2 and 3, 1909 meeting of the regents there was a statement that twelve members of the university faculty, including Stoops, Jansky, and Williams, "failed of re-election" at the June, 1908 meeting of the regents held in Oklahoma City. These 1908 minutes have not been located.

September, 1909, lists nine members of the faculty of the school, including professors Bobo, Capshaw, DeBarr, Lane, Maclaren, Turley, Washburn, and Guy Y. Williams. John Chester Darling, M.S., was the ninth faculty member; he was physical director with the rank of associate professor. Anatomy courses were taught by professors Capshaw and Turley, chemistry by professors DeBarr and Williams, and pathology by Professor Turley. Professor Washburn, who became dean of the School of Pharmacy in 1909, taught only pharmaceutical methods, while Professor Maclaren taught physiology, pharmacology, materia medica, and therapeutics. Professor Lane's teaching was limited to medical embryology. Concerning faculty salaries for the biennium July, 1909, to June, 1911, professors received $1,500 to $2,500; associate professors, $1,500 to $2,150; and assistant professors, $1,000 to $1,350. The state appropriations to the entire university for the 1909–11 biennium were approximately $153,190 a year. Starting in 1909 the fiscal agency for the university was the state board of affairs.

The official university records reported sixteen students enrolled in the School of Medicine in the year 1908–1909. According to the *American Medical Directory* for 1909, there was no tuition charge for students. The June, 1909, catalog and the September, 1909, bulletin for the School of Medicine announced, "Students who complete the first 2 years of medicine may receive not to exceed 64 hours credit toward the degree of Bachelor of Science unqualified in the College of Arts and Sciences."

It is interesting that the peak number of physicians in Oklahoma was reached soon after statehood, the result of a great influx of doctors from other states. In 1909 there were 2,703 physicians in the state, an average of one to each 587 persons.[8]

It is not surprising that the School of Medicine made little progress during the turbulent first years of statehood. This was a period of recoil from territorial government and swashbuckling political controversy and a time of progressive changes, as well as perplexity, for the state colleges. Governor Haskell officiated with energy and daring, recommending action on bank stabilization,

[8] Litton, *History of Oklahoma*, 380–81.

the initiative and referendum, regulation of trusts and monopolies, and prohibition. The first legislature (1907–1909), in the spirit of reform, was the busiest in state history in dealing with the above matters, as well as with labor, safety, and health and sanitation codes. A corporation commission, bank guaranty law, and a graduated income tax were initiated—also a Jim Crow Code. In the field of education, advance was chiefly in regard to the public school system. The second legislature (1909–10) was concerned heavily with distributing the major state institutions.

In 1910 the Carnegie Foundation completed *Medical Education in the United States and Canada*, a survey of medical schools, also known as the *Flexner Report*. The survey had a momentous impact on medical education in the United States. Dr. Arthur Dean Bevan recounted the role of the Council on Medical Education in this memorable and historic project. "Fifty schools agreed to require by 1910 or before, at least one year of university physics, chemistry, and biology, and one modern language as a preliminary education before matriculating in medicine. Immediately a number of consolidations were arranged in many cities having several schools.

"It early became apparent that as soon as the one year and then the two year university requirement of physics, chemistry, and biology were generally adopted, homeopathy and eclecticism would die for the lack of students and this proved to be the case.

"Rapidly the better medical schools sought affiliation with universities, and after the most part became in fact University Medical Departments. Gradually the University has exerted more and more influence on and control of medical education and this is most fortunate. It would, however, be unfortunate if this control was ever used to exclude the influence and control that should be exerted on medical education by the medical profession.

"As the work of the council [the Council on Medical Education] developed, it occurred to some of the members of the council that if we could obtain the publication and approval of our work by the Carnegie Foundation for the Advancement of Teaching, it would assist materially in securing the results we were attempting to bring about. With this in mind we approached President Henry S. Pritchett of the Carnegie Foundation and presented to him the evidence we had accumulated and asked him to make it the subject of a special report on medical education to be published by the Carnegie Foundation. He enthusiastically agreed to this proposition."[9]

The *Carnegie Foundation Report on Medical Education in the United States and Canada* (also known as the *Flexner Report*), by Abraham Flexner, was published in the spring of 1910. It came at a most opportune time to help, and help very materially, in the big task which the American Medical Association had undertaken of evaluating the standards of medical education in this country and of placing the American medical schools on a sound basis.

This survey was begun in January, 1909. Visits to 155 existing medical schools (147 in the United States and 8 in Canada) were made by Dr. N. P. Colwell and Abraham Flexner. The second inspection of the University of Oklahoma School of Medicine was made on November 12, 1909.[10] By the time of the report, which rated the University of Oklahoma School of Medicine as acceptable, the number of medical schools had been reduced to 126. There were 61 four-year schools and 11 other two-year medical schools with a similar rating in the survey.[11]

In 1910 the entrance requirement for medical schools, as given by the Council on Medical Education, was completion of a four-year high school education or its equivalent, whereas that of the Association of Southern Medical Colleges required only two years of preparatory school or high school, or its equivalent.

---

9 Bevan, "Cooperation in Medical Education and Medical Service," *Journal of the American Medical Association*, Vol. XC (1928), 1173.

10 Abraham Flexner, *I Remember* (New York, Simon and Schuster, 1940), 129.

11 *Journal of the American Medical Association*, Vol. LV (1910), 693. Brief documents filed by Dean Patterson on March 27 and July 8, 1939, entitled "History of the University of Oklahoma School of Medicine and Its Teaching Hospitals," state erroneously that the School of Medicine was first inspected by Dr. Colwell for the Council on Medical Education in 1909, and that it was accorded what is known as a class B rating in 1910 because of the lack of controlled teaching facilities. See also Patterson, "Medical School has 964 Graduates," *Sooner Magazine*, Vol. XI (August 7, 1939), 27.

At the turn of the century there had been several attempts to establish medical schools in Oklahoma Territory, apart from the university School of Medicine founded in 1900 at Norman. All of these schools,[12] with the exception of one in Guthrie, were in Oklahoma City, and all except the Epworth University College of Medicine and its successor turned out to be futile ventures.

According to the *American Medical Directory* for 1909, the Twentieth Century Physiomedical College was organized at Guthrie, Oklahoma, in 1900. Its charter was revoked in 1904, on the basis that it was a fraudulent school which advertised certificates for a fee of ten dollars apiece.[13]

The 1902 *Journal of the American Medical Association* states: "Oklahoma may have one medical college in the immediate future. A charter has been obtained, a partial faculty of eighteen selected, and plans laid to open the school on October 1."[14] The name of this school was the Oklahoma City Medical College. It was sponsored by a group of Oklahoma City physicians at a time when the city had a population of 10,037 and two hospitals with an aggregate of one hundred beds. The *Oklahoma Medical News-Journal* for May, 1902, announced that a charter had been granted and that a fifteen-thousand dollar building was being planned. Dr. John H. Threadgill was the president; Dr. G. A. Wall, the dean; and Dr. W. T. Salmon, the secretary-treasurer of the Oklahoma City Medical College. Those officers signified their intention of following the regulations of the Association of American Medical Colleges in administering the school.

The twenty-two member faculty of the Oklahoma City Medical College included Professor Edwin DeBarr, Dr. W. E. Dicken, Dr. John W. Duke, Dr. R. T. Edwards, Dr. John A. Reck, Dr. Joseph B. Rolater, Dr. W. T. Salmon, Dr. Delos Walker, Dr. G. A. Wall, Dr. Archa K. West, and Dr. C. W. Williams. Edwin DeBarr was

[12] Twentieth Century Physiomedical College, 1900; Oklahoma City Medical College, 1902–1903; Epworth University College of Medicine, 1904–1907; the first Oklahoma State Medical College, 1905; the second Oklahoma State Medical College, 1907; Oklahoma Medical College, 1907–1909; and Epworth College of Medicine, 1907–10.

[13] *Journal of the American Medical Association*, Vol. XLIII (1904), 990.

[14] *Journal of the American Medical Association*, Vol. XXXIX (1902), 567.

already professor of chemistry at the University of Oklahoma, and later Dr. West, Dr. Duke, Dr. Reck, and Dr. Rolater joined the faculty of the University of Oklahoma School of Medicine. All of the physicians named above maintained their interest in medical education and subsequently served on one or more faculties of the Epworth College of Medicine, the Oklahoma Medical College, or the Southwest Postgraduate Medical College. The Oklahoma City Medical College apparently never instituted active teaching, since the *Journal of the American Medical Association* reported "Oklahoma school not yet in operation."[15]

On August 24, 1905, the *Daily Oklahoman* announced that Dr. N. G. Weeks, of Chicago, was filing articles of incorporation for a medical college, to be constructed in the Aurora Addition of Oklahoma City, at a cost of $75,000. Apparently this school, to have been named the Oklahoma State Medical College, never was built.

On February 17, 1907, the *Daily Oklahoman* carried another announcement, that articles of incorporation for another Oklahoma State Medical College, in Oklahoma City, had been filed with State Secretary Filson. The incorporators and stockholders included a number of prominent physicians, among them Dr. W. J. Darnell, of Mountain View, president; Dr. J. R. Phelan, of Oklahoma City, secretary; Dr. West Moreland, actually William Westmoreland, of Atlanta, Georgia; Dr. H. H. Battey, of Rome, Georgia; and J. P. Eckers, of Oklahoma City. Dr. Westmoreland was a professor of surgery in the Atlanta College of Physicians and Surgeons, a past vice-president of the American Medical Association, and ex-president of the Georgia State Medical Association. With reference to the proposed Oklahoma State Medical College, Dr. Phelan was quoted as saying, "It will be conducted as a regular medical college. It will open for a four year course beginning next September. During the next four weeks the cost and site of a college building will be determined." This medical school evidently never reached an operational stage.

Another school of short duration, the Oklahoma Medical Col-

[15] *Journal of the American Medical Association*, Vol. XLI (1903), 451.

lege, opened in Oklahoma City in 1907. Dr. Gregory A. Wall was president, Dr. William T. Salmon was dean, and Dr. Thomas A. Buchanan was secretary.[16] In addition there were thirty-two other Oklahoma City physicians on the faculty, including Dr. J. W. Duke and Dr. Delos Walker, mentioned on the Oklahoma City Medical College faculty; Dr. W. A. Fullington and V. G. Shinkle, B.S., who were also on the Epworth College of Medicine faculty; and F. J. Bolend, Ph.C., Dr. Gayfree Ellison, and Dr. W. M. Taylor, all of whom later joined the University of Oklahoma School of Medicine faculty. Dr. E. S. Lain, also on the faculty of the Oklahoma Medical College, was subsequently on the faculties of the Epworth College of Medicine, the University of Oklahoma School of Medicine, and the Southwest Postgraduate Medical College.

The second annual session of the Oklahoma Medical College was described in its bulletin for the year 1908–1909. The cost of room and board at that time was given as three to five dollars a week. Plans for a school building were outlined, though the building was never erected. The faculty members of the Oklahoma Medical College taught in St. Anthony and Rolater hospitals. In the previous year there had been only three students in the school. In 1909, though the school had adopted the requirements of the Association of American Medical Colleges, it received a C rating and was terminated.

A more successful venture was the organization, in Oklahoma City, of a college of medicine in 1904 by Epworth University.[17] On July 6, 1904, the Epworth University Board of Trustees elected a general faculty for the university and, at the same time, appointed the following faculty members for its College of Medicine: Drs. Archa K. West, H. Coulter Todd, Lea A. Riely, U. L. Russell, F. C. Hoops, J. A. Ryan, and William J. Jolly. This faculty elected Dr.

16 These officials are named in an advertisement in the December, 1907 issue of the *Oklahoma Medical News-Journal*. In earlier August and September advertisements Dr. J. R. Phelan was listed as dean and Dr. Y. E. Colville was listed as secretary. An interim advertisement in October indicates that Dr. G. A. Wall was the secretary.

17 For an official history of the Epworth College of Medicine, see H. Coulter Todd, "History of Medical Education in Oklahoma from 1904 to 1910," *Bulletin of the University of Oklahoma*, University Studies, No. 26 (1928), 13–28.

West as dean and Dr. Todd as secretary. The College of Medicine opened with three students in attendance, increasing to seven students during the remainder of the 1904–1905 session. Classes were held in the new Epworth University building until 1907. The *Journal of the American Medical Association* included the Epworth University College of Medicine in its 1904 list of medical schools.

In 1905–1906 the faculty had been increased to nineteen members. Dr. Todd, in his history, states that the faculty members were pioneers in medical education who received no compensation for the service spent in the effort to build a reputable medical school and that indeed many were struggling to make a livelihood at the same time. Due to inadequate hospital facilities for medical education—since there was no such thing as a teaching hospital, they had to use private patients for instruction. Furthermore, teaching was handicapped by the territorial laws which made it difficult to obtain dissecting material.

On the brighter side, Oklahoma City was experiencing a major boom, and a number of highly trained physicians who had come to the city possessed a determination to make it a center of medical learning. Consequently the *Daily Oklahoman* for April 7, 1905, states: "The Medical College of Epworth University has been organized as a permanent department with a full four year course. A building is to be erected for a laboratory and dissecting room, a hospital for clinical work, and a nurses training school. The executive committee of Epworth University met in Mr. C. B. Ames' office. Twenty medical faculty members were named; they are planning for the erection of a building on the university campus. There was discussion of the Oklahoma City Hospital (formerly the Protestant Hospital) as possibly becoming a part of the medical school for clinical teaching."

During the year 1906–1907 the curriculum of the Medical College of Epworth University was built up to a total of almost four thousand hours, and a full four-year course was instituted. In 1907 the school became a separate corporation, named the Epworth College of Medicine, which was listed as a member of the Southern Medical College Association from 1907 to 1909.[18] Members of the corporation included nineteen physicians who purchased and remodeled the Angelo Hotel at the northwest corner of Sixth and North Broadway Streets for a sum of nineteen thousand dollars. This structure had twenty-three rooms and a dining room. Dr. L. H. Buxton was president of the corporation, and Dr. E. S. Ferguson was secretary. No salaries were ever paid to the faculty members. Advertisements in the *Oklahoma Medical News-Journal*, during 1907, claimed that the college had excellent laboratories and large clinics. The Council on Medical Education inspected the Epworth College of Medicine in 1907. The college was given a C or unacceptable rating which was continued through the remainder of its existence.

Faculty members for the years 1905–10 are listed in Dr. Todd's history. During 1907–1908 there were twenty-three faculty members and a student body of twenty-three. Dr. Antonio D. Young became the secretary of the faculty that year. In the 1908–1909 academic year there were thirty-one faculty members and a student body of twenty. Apparently there were forty-one faculty members during 1909–10, the last year of the Epworth College of Medicine, although Dr. Todd in his history names only thirty-nine. According to Roy Gittinger, Dr. Everett S. Lain and Dr. Joseph T. Martin were also members, making a total of forty-one.[19] Also Dr. Lain, in a personal communication, affirmed that he was a member of the faculty at that time.

An appraisal of the faculty of the Epworth College of Medicine indicates that the basic science teaching in this school, from 1907 to 1910, was contributed by local practicing physicians, with the exception of James W. Mayberry, M.S. who was professor of chemistry during the year 1908–10 and Dr. J. M. Finney, who

---

[18] In 1911, Epworth University was moved to Guthrie and renamed the Oklahoma Methodist University. In 1919 it returned to Oklahoma City under its present name, Oklahoma City University.

[19] Gittinger, *The University of Oklahoma*, 65.

taught part of the anatomy course during 1908–10. There were forty-seven students in the college during the last year.[20]

The report *Medical Education in the United States and Canada* (the *Flexner Report*) included the Epworth College of Medicine by name under the following aspects of the critique: "Some of the very worst [medical schools] are known as University departments. . . . It stretches terms to speak of laboratory teaching. . . . Institutions that lend their name to proprietary medical schools for which they can do nothing and which they cannot control . . . ."[21] Specific inadequacies stated for the Epworth College of Medicine were that clinical instruction was in a hospital having only thirty to forty beds available for instruction and that the majority of the cases were surgical ones; that the laboratory facilities were nominal, disorderly, and neglected; and that there was no dispensary provision. One author suggests that the college did have a dispensary on Reno Street in 1905.[22] It may have been discontinued prior to the report.

The *Flexner Report* made the following recommendations concerning medical education in the state: "Oklahoma might well support the work of the first two years on a much more liberal basis. It would be advisable for the State University of Oklahoma to engage in clinical work in Oklahoma City. Oklahoma may from Norman govern a medical school in Oklahoma City. The new commonwealth of Oklahoma may, if wise, avoid most of the evils which this report has described, for though they have already appeared, they have not taken deep root. Immigration of physicians, among

[20] For a complete list of the sixteen graduates of Epworth College of Medicine, 1907–10, see Gittinger, *The University of Oklahoma*, 201.

[21] The author finds no basis in the *Flexner Report* for the misleading statement made in *Today's Health*, Vol. XLVII (March, 1969), 70, that "It was, after all, rather shattering to read that the Epworth College of Medicine in Oklahoma City . . . was nothing more than a profitable stock company for a few individuals." Also, in the *Journal of the Oklahoma State Medical Association*, Vol. XX (1927), 176, Dr. H. Coulter Todd states, "In 1906 . . . the rapidly growing Epworth College of Medicine . . . affiliated with St. Anthony and the City Hospital for clinical instruction . . . . Not one of these doctors connected with Epworth ever received one cent for the services he rendered, all the tuition received being put back into equipment for teaching."

[22] Basil Hayes, *Leroy Long, Teacher of Medicine*, (Oklahoma City, privately printed, 1943).

others, has been so rapid that the State has easily three times as many doctors as it needs. They pour in from the schools of St. Louis, Kansas City and Chicago. If however, the state wishes a high grade supply only, it must speedily define standards such as will suppress commercial schools, as for example that now nominally belonging to Epworth University, and by the same action exclude inferior doctors trained elsewhere. Having done this, only an institution with considerable resources derived either from taxes or from endowment will even attempt to conduct a medical school in the state, which is as it should be. The State University is of course marked out for the work. Its present modest beginning must be developed. Perhaps it will have at once to occupy Oklahoma City with a clinical department, so as to obtain control of the field."

The Epworth College of Medicine was terminated in 1910. The property which it owned was sold for thirty thousand dollars, after reverting to the corporation, which was then dissolved. The closing of this college should be considered with a certain degree of sympathetic understanding. It had become a hopeless task for groups of physicians without financial assistance or guidance from any institution or government agency to operate a reputable medical school that could meet the standards set up at that time. Nevertheless, the sincere and active interest of some of the practicing physicians in the development of medical education in Oklahoma and elsewhere in the nation has been an impressive phenomenon (see Appendix II).

The work of Abraham Flexner and of the Council on Medical Education exerted a profound influence upon medical education throughout the country. In Oklahoma the *Flexner Report* marked the end of the ten-year span of attempts by physicians to establish proprietary schools of medicine in the state. The only additional medical college to come into existence subsequently was the Southwest Postgraduate Medical College, which was founded in Oklahoma City in 1911.

IV. The Organization of the Four-Year School of Medicine: 1910

THE YEAR 1910 marks the beginning of the four-year program at the School of Medicine of the University of Oklahoma and the end of the Epworth College of Medicine in Oklahoma City.

According to a brief note dictated by Dr. L. A. Turley in 1938, there had been an agreement between the regents of the university and the Epworth College of Medicine to accept into the university the students then attending the Epworth College of Medicine, allowing them to proceed with their medical education. In consideration of this action, the Epworth College of Medicine agreed to dissolve. Dr. Turley further stated that the stockholders of the Epworth College of Medicine retained all property belonging to them.

A somewhat more detailed account appeared in the report from the university to E. D. Cameron, state superintendent of public instruction, concerning the period from statehood to June 30, 1910: "Extension of medical work—In the spring of 1910 negotiations with the Regents of the University were opened by the faculty and stockholders of the Epworth College of Medicine in Oklahoma City. They desired to relinquish the work which they had been doing for about five years, provided some arrangements could be made for giving third and fourth year medical work in Oklahoma City. They proposed that if the Regents of the University would provide for this work, they would so far as possible transfer their students and hand over this work to the State University. After full discussion of the matter the Regents decided that it would be best to take this work, and make the best provision which seemed possible for the coming year. The members of the faculty of the former Epworth College of Medicine volunteered their services as professors and instructors for third and fourth year work and they undertook collectively to assume all responsibility for the expenses of carrying on this work during the year 1910 to 1911.[1] Under the arrangement thus consummated the University of Oklahoma has a complete medical school, the first two years work being done at Norman, and the last two years in Oklahoma City. The clinical faculty in Oklahoma City has rented a building[2] for classwork which is convenient and sufficient for the present needs of the school. The authorities in charge of the hospitals in Oklahoma City have cooperated very readily with the new School of Medicine and we find that abundant opportunity for clinical work is furnished by them."

The minutes of the first State Regents of the University of Oklahoma indicate that on March 8, 1910, Dr. L. Haynes Buxton, president of the Board of Directors of the Epworth College of Medicine, appeared and addressed the regents upon the matter of the university taking over the Epworth College of Medicine.

At the same meeting President Evans presented a report: "The School of Medicine has made a substantial advance in its enrollment during the year, practically doubling any that it has had before. Overtures have been made during the year and especially during the last few weeks by the Epworth College of Medicine for us to arrange some method by which we could take over their work, receiving such first and second year students as they can send to us here, and making provision for the work of the third and fourth years in Oklahoma City where they can have the hos-

---

1 Pertinent to this arrangement is the following abstract from a 1910 statute relative to the authority of the Board of Regents of the University of Oklahoma: ". . . the board of regents are hereby authorized to establish such professional and other colleges or departments when in their judgment they may be deemed necessary and proper: Provided that no money shall be expended by the board of regents in establishing and organizing any of the additional colleges or departments provided for in this section until an appropriation therefor shall have first been made." The third legislature did not come into session until January, 1911, five months after the start of the school year.

2 The building was located at N.W. Tenth and Lee Streets.

pital and clinical advantages necessary for this work. I attended the American Medical Association [meeting] during February and was pleased to learn from the reports given there that our work so far as it goes is placed in the highest class.

"The Epworth College has been unable, with the facilities at its command, to do standard work, especially in the first two years. I have hesitated about taking any step which might even have the appearance of trying to take from Epworth University any of its work. I am assured, however, by members of the faculty of the Epworth College of Medicine, that it is an altogether separate corporation, that it feels it has not the facilities for doing standard work, especially in the first two years, and that while it has a number of men able and willing to give third and fourth year instruction practically freely, it has no men who feel that they can spare their time and energy for the administrative work of such a college. They therefore ask that we should consider making some arrangement with them by which the two last years of their course can be developed into the completion of our own medical school.

"I have stated that in my judgment we can not formally undertake work, at least work involving any expenditure of funds outside of Norman, without special act of the Legislature. As it seems fully decided that their work must be abandoned if no arrangements can be made at once, I have suggested that the Regents might be asked to consider the proposition that the faculties of our school and the Epworth College should be asked to hold a joint meeting and agree upon an absolutely standard four year course of instruction, that the University School of Medicine should give its course just as it has done, giving the first two years of this course, that the faculty of the Epworth College of Medicine should make provision for carrying on during the next year the work of the last two years with the understanding that a recommendation should be made as strongly as possible to the next Legislature to allow this work to be reorganized as a part of the work of the University School of Medicine. If this arrangement is made we should have at once to make a careful estimate of the additional expense likely

46

to be involved in this, and until the Legislature acts it would have to be understood that the expense of maintaining the work in Oklahoma City will have to be met either by tuition or in some other way by those interested in the work in that city.

"It seems to me also that if this work is to be undertaken we must take steps at once to find out from the people of Oklahoma City what suggestions can be made as to a location for such buildings as may be necessary for the part of the work of this school to be done there."

The question was discussed at length by members of the board. It was moved and seconded that a committee of board members and the president of the university be appointed and empowered to take this matter up with the Epworth College of Medicine. If, after investigation, they found the university able to locate the third and fourth years of the medical department at Oklahoma City, they were to make the necessary arrangements. Otherwise the committee was to enter into such correlation with Epworth College of Medicine as would lead eventually to the unification of the two schools. The motion was carried. President Cruce then appointed Nathaniel Lee Linebaugh, Claude C. Hatchett, William Eugene Rowsey, and President Evans to the committee.

The *Daily Oklahoman* of Wednesday, March 9, had nothing to say of what had transpired at the meeting of the board of regents other than that they had met and that their president, Lee Cruce, had given the annual report. However, a story did appear in the Monday, March 14, edition of the same newspaper, entitled: "Epworth Medics Strong for Union—Parade Street, Giving Endorsement of Plan to Merge Medical Colleges," which read, in part, as follows:

"Armed with megaphones, bedecked with ribbons, flying pennants, and a complement of yells guaranteed to raise the dead, a bunch of Epworth medical students took the day off Saturday, and paraded the streets of Oklahoma City in a demonstration calculated to express their hearty endorsement of the proposed plan to amalgamate the medical schools of Epworth and Oklahoma Universities into one strong institution known as the Epworth State

Medical School, two years of work being done at Norman and the last two in Oklahoma City, where clinics are plentiful.

"After completely subduing the business districts, the celebrating students boarded street cars and went for the conquest of the residence portions of the city fastening their banners to the backs of cars, and hanging from the windows."

A report in the *Daily Oklahoman*, on Thursday, April 13, 1910, concerning another meeting of the regents, stated only that they had reelected Dr. Bobo as dean of the School of Medicine whose "third and fourth years are at Oklahoma City." His duties were increased, and a salary of fifteen hundred dollars per annum was allowed.

However, the minutes show that other items of business were considered. It is on record that the following petition, dated March 17, 1910, was presented from the Epworth College of Medicine: "To the Board of Regents, University of Oklahoma. We the undersigned Board of Directors of the corporation, the Epworth College of Medicine, hereby make application to become a part of the University of Oklahoma. The dissolution of the above mentioned corporation is now pending and the same will be consummated as soon as legally possible.

> Respectfully, L. Haynes Buxton, President
> A. K. West, Dean
> M. Smith, Vice-President
> Antonio D. Young, Secretary
> Lea A. Riely, Treasurer"[3]

A report of the regents' Committee on the Medical School was then read, recommending that the university absorb the former

[3] In the Wednesday, March 23 issue of the *Daily Oklahoman* there appeared an article entitled, "Medical School is to Dissolve." It stated that the "dissolution papers for Epworth College of Medicine were filed in the district court Tuesday by five members of the Board of Directors of the school (Drs. L. H. Buxton, Lea Riely, M. Smith, A. K. West, and A. D. Young). At a meeting of the stockholders on Monday, March 14, the motion for this action was carried. The entire amount of capital stock is $20,000. The personal property is valued at $500. It is generally supposed that this step is taken so that no complications will arise when the medical school of the state is united with Epworth."

Epworth College of Medicine and that the third and fourth years of medicine be located at Oklahoma City. A motion that the report be adopted, that the application for absorption be accepted, and that part of the School of Medicine be located as recommended was carried. A list of the proposed faculty was presented; this faculty was officially adopted.

Finally, in a letter to Dean Robert Patterson in 1938, F. E. Cargill, manager for the *American Medical Directory*, stated: "This incorporated stock company (the Epworth College of Medicine) disbanded May 5, 1910, and the remains of the Epworth College of Medicine merged by affiliation with the State University of Oklahoma School of Medicine, Norman and Oklahoma City." Both the Council on Medical Education and the Association of American Medical Colleges had approved this merger.

Some other factors relative to the merger are discussed by Dr. H. C. Todd. "The task of operating the [rapidly growing] school [Epworth College of Medicine] was naturally becoming a great burden to the men who had already given so much of their time and effort. . . . A committee composed of Drs. L. Haynes Buxton, A. K. West, and H. Coulter Todd was named to confer with the authorities of the University of Oklahoma, in 1910, to ascertain if the Epworth College of Medicine could not be affiliated with or taken over by the University of Oklahoma.

"These were years fraught with disappointments and difficulties but the men in back of this Epworth College of Medicine were men of high ideals and had but one purpose, namely to build up a creditable medical school in Oklahoma. How well they succeeded is proved by the fact that they were able to turn over to the State University over twenty trained medical teachers, and a student body numbering forty seven."[4]

The 1910 *Educational Number of the Journal of the American Medical Association* listed the University of Oklahoma School of Medicine as a four-year school which offered the M.D. degree and,

4 Todd, "The History of Medical Education in Oklahoma from 1904 to 1910," *Bulletin of the University of Oklahoma, University Studies*, No. 26 (1928), 25.

upon completion of a six-year course, both a B.S. degree and an M.D. degree.[5]

The university did acquire the services of some of the clinicians who had previously taught at the Epworth College of Medicine, and, in keeping with the agreement, assumed its obligations to the students transferring from that school. The School of Medicine of the university continued to conduct its first two years of instruction at the main university campus in Norman and instituted its third and fourth clinical years in Oklahoma City in the fall of 1910. The expanded faculty consisted of twenty-seven professors and twelve instructors. The combined student enrollment in June, 1910, was seventy-two. This number was reduced to sixty-three by the close of the 1910–11 academic year. Prior to the merger, twenty-one students had enrolled at the University of Oklahoma School of Medicine in Norman for the academic year 1909–10.[6] The student fees were set as follows: first year, $30; second year, $10; third year, $100; fourth year, $105.

Concerning the clinical facilities for work in the third and fourth years, the June, 1910, catalog of the university explained: "The work is done in the hospitals and clinical laboratories of Oklahoma City. Seven hospitals and three out-patient departments furnish a daily average of over three hundred cases of human illness or injury which are acceptable to the faculty and students for use in studying the science of disease and the art of healing."

The newly expanded University of Oklahoma School of Medicine continued as a member of the Association of American Medical Colleges and as an acceptable class A school as it faced new and challenging responsibilities.

[5] *Journal of the American Medical Association, Educational Number*, Vol. LV (1910), 674.

[6] For a list of the fifty-three former students enrolled in the two-year medical course at Norman prior to 1910, see *Bulletin of the University of Oklahoma School of Medicine*, New Series, No. 36 (June, 1910), 43. Included in the list are Walter L. Capshaw, John Chester Darling, Fenton M. Sanger, and Roscoe Walker, all of whom later became members of the faculty of the University of Oklahoma School of Medicine. There were seven graduates of the Epworth College of Medicine in 1910. For a list of the sixteen graduates from Epworth, 1907–10, see *Bulletin of the University of Oklahoma School of Medicine*, New Series, No. 36 (June, 1910), 46. Among them were Dr. Fenton M. Sanger, Dr. Marvin Stout, and Drs. Walter and Eva Wells.

50

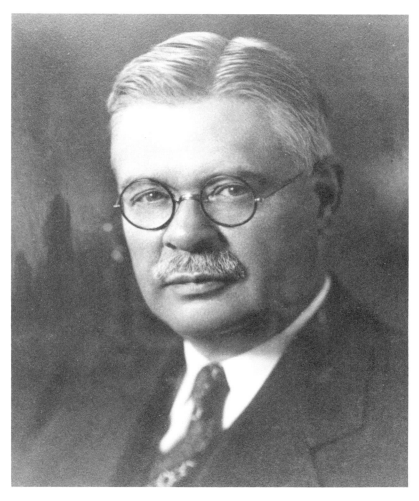

In 1900, Lawrence N. Upjohn, M.D., was appointed director of the premedical department at the University of Oklahoma, a two-year medical course which was the first medical school organized in Oklahoma Territory.

Courtesy University of Oklahoma Medical Center

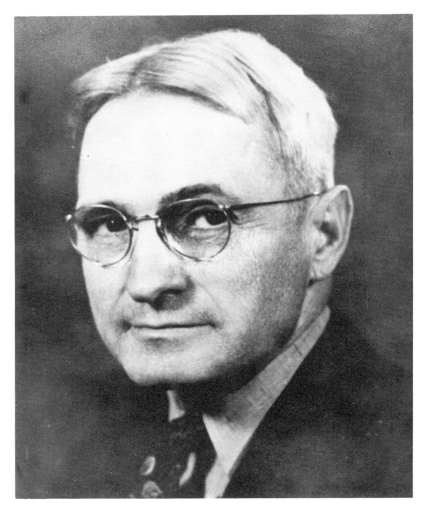

Roy Philson Stoops, M.D., succeeded Dr. Upjohn as director of the medical department in 1904. In 1907 his title was changed to acting dean.

Courtesy University of Oklahoma Medical Center

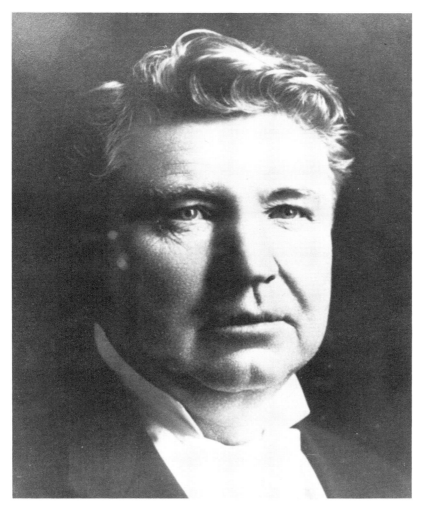

Charles Sharp Bobo, M.D., head of the Department of Forensic Medicine, 1906–10, and dean of the School of Medicine, 1908–11.

Courtesy University of Oklahoma Medical Center

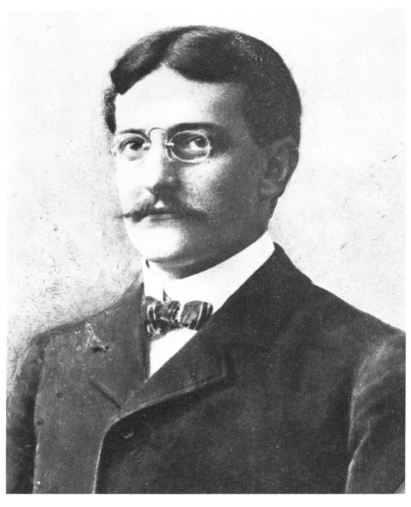

Robert Findlater Williams, M.D., dean of the School of Medicine, 1911–13.

Courtesy University of Oklahoma Medical Center

54

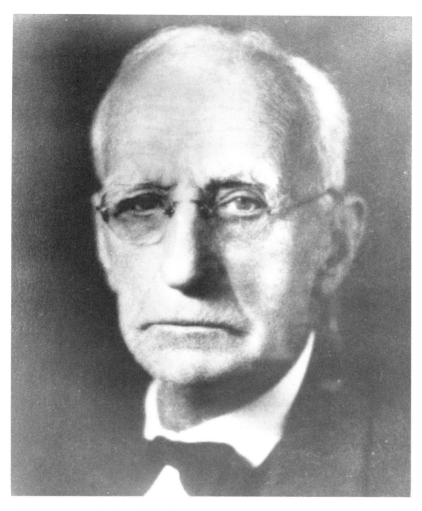

William James Jolly, M.D., head of the Department of Surgery, 1912–13, and acting dean of the School of Medicine, 1913.

Courtesy University of Oklahoma Medical Center

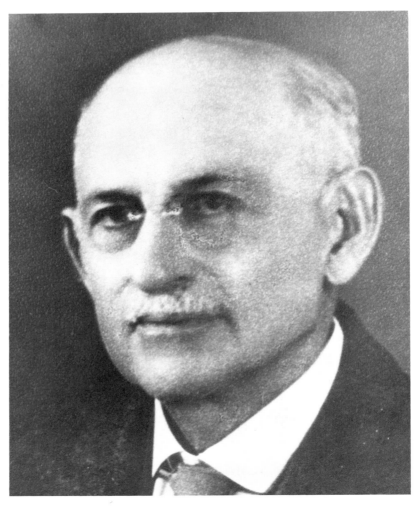

Curtis Richard Day, M.D., head of the Department of Urology, 1911–13, and dean of the School of Medicine, 1914–15.

Courtesy University of Oklahoma Medical Center

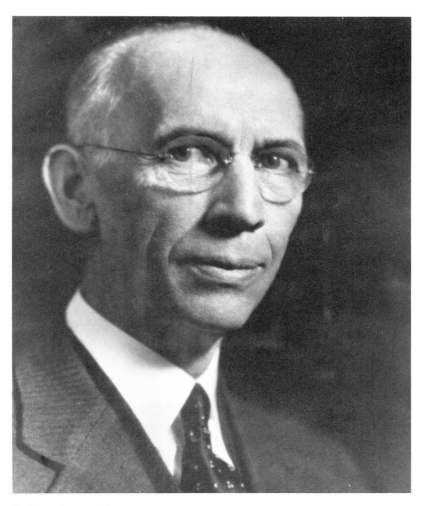

LeRoy Long, M.D., served as dean of the School of Medicine from 1915 to 1931. Under his guidance the School of Medicine once again received a class A rating, and the University Hospital became a reality. He was also head of the Department of Surgery, 1915–31.

Courtesy University of Oklahoma Medical Center

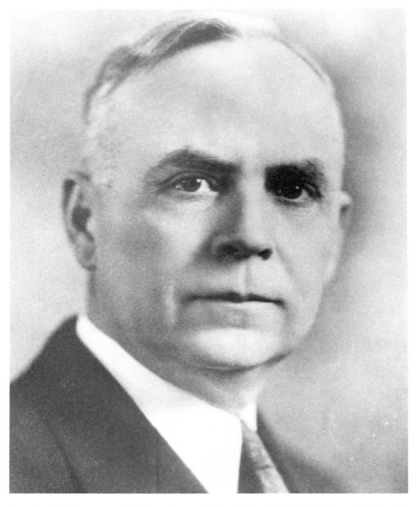

Lewis J. Moorman, M.D., dean of the School of Medicine, 1931–35.

Courtesy University of Oklahoma Medical Center

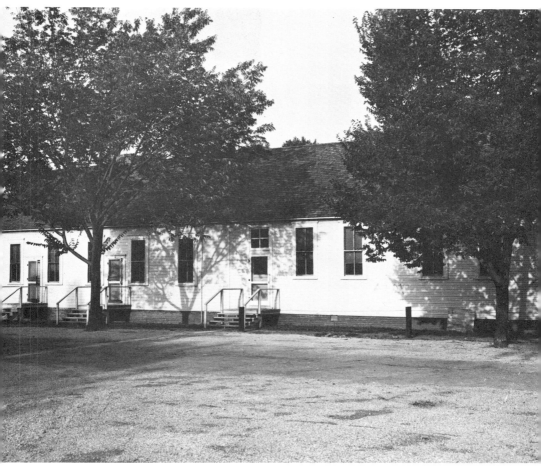

This frame building, constructed in 1900 to house the Department of Anatomy on the university campus in Norman, was the first structure in Oklahoma Territory designed exclusively for medical teaching.

Courtesy Sooner Medic

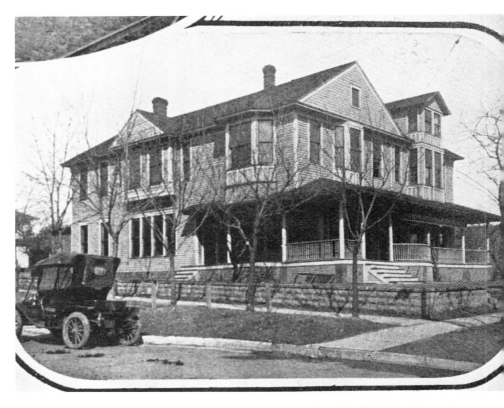

The Epworth College of Medicine was organized in 1904 by Epworth University. In 1910, Epworth College merged with the University of Oklahoma School of Medicine to establish a four-year medical course.

Courtesy Oklahoma County Main Library

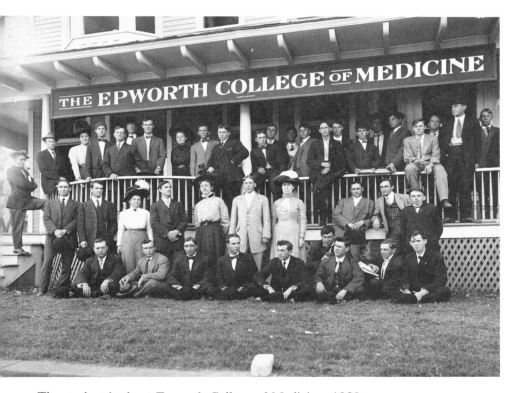

The student body at Epworth College of Medicine, 1909.

Courtesy Dr. Blair Points

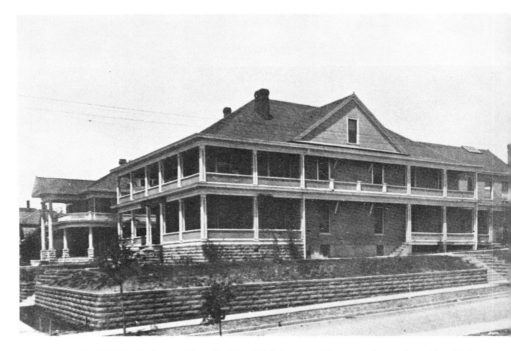

In 1911, Rolater Hospital in Oklahoma City was leased to the University of Oklahoma as a hospital and quarters for the School of Medicine.

Courtesy Oklahoma County Main Library

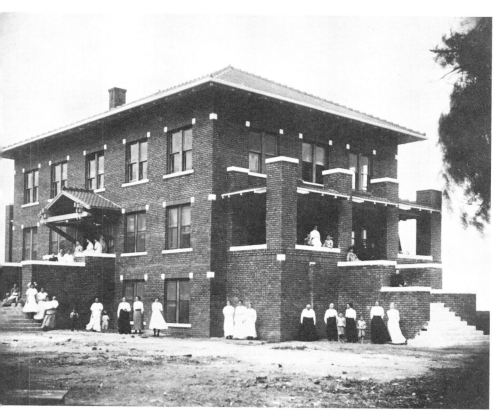

Holmes Home of Redeeming Love, established in 1900 in Guthrie, Oklahoma, by the Free Methodist Church of North America, moved to Oklahoma City in 1910, where it extended teaching privileges to the University of Oklahoma School of Medicine.

Courtesy Deaconess Hospital

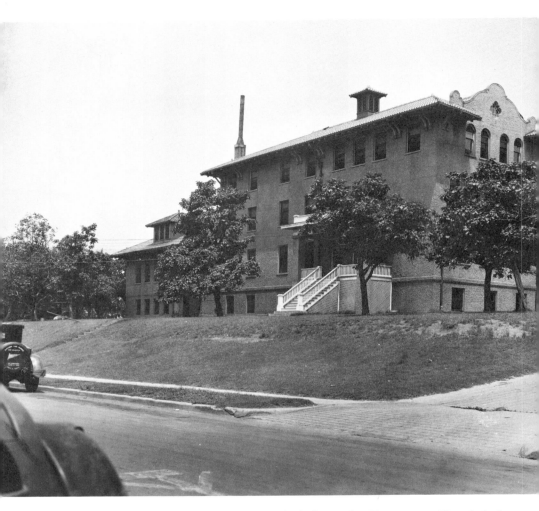

Southwest Postgraduate Hospital, later the Emergency Hospital, in Oklahoma City.

Courtesy Sooner Medic

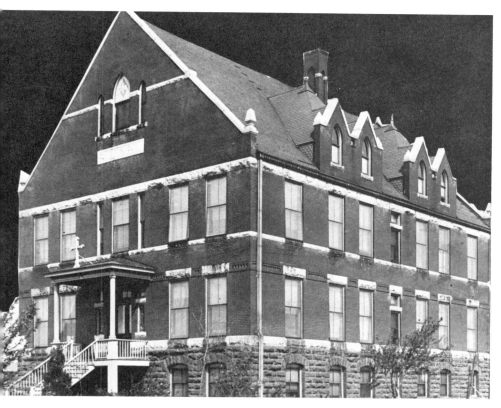

St. Anthony Hospital in Oklahoma City, pictured here in 1899, also
extended teaching privileges to the University of Oklahoma School of
Medicine.

Courtesy Oklahoma Historical Society

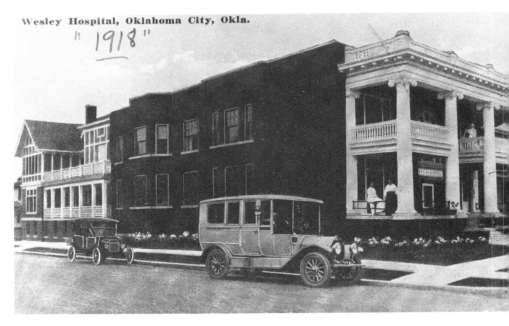

Wesley Hospital in Oklahoma City, 1918.

Courtesy Presbyterian Hospital

One of the immediate needs was to move the offices of the dean of the University of Oklahoma School of Medicine from Norman to Oklahoma City. Dr. Charles S. Bobo, dean of the School of Medicine at the time, with the aid of Dr. A. K. West, who had been dean of the Epworth College of Medicine and was now professor of medicine at the university, organized the clinical teaching program that began in Oklahoma City in the fall of 1910. The arrangements for the opening on September 16 of the four-year school were completed under the direction of Professor John D. Maclaren, secretary of the School of Medicine. The *Daily Oklahoman* of August 28, 1910, anticipating the formal beginning, stated: "It will open with an address by A. Grant Evans, President. The opening exercises will be held in the building at N. W. Tenth and Lee Streets, which will be the permanent headquarters of the institution."

Dean Bobo organized a medical council consisting of Professors Abraham L. Blesh, Walter L. Capshaw, Robert M. Howard, John D. Maclaren, Louis A. Turley, and Archa K. West. A clinical advisory board included Professors Blesh, Howard, and West. Bobo also appointed a committee on medical curriculum—Professors Maclaren, Lea A. Riely, and Antonio D. Young.

It is appropriate to reflect here upon the lives of the three Epworth faculty members, Drs. Buxton, Todd, and West, who made the initial proposal for the formation of a four-year university School of Medicine and who contributed energetically to its fulfillment.

Dr. Lauren Haynes Buxton, M.D., LL.D., was an important leader in the founding of the Epworth College of Medicine and in its subsequent merger into the University of Oklahoma. He was born in Vermont, in 1859, and graduated from the medical department of the University of Vermont in 1884. He had been an eye, ear, nose, and throat specialist before coming to Guthrie, Oklahoma, to practice medicine. In 1899, he moved to Oklahoma City. From 1897 to 1900, Dr. Buxton was territorial superintendent of public health; from 1897 to 1901, he was secretary of the Territorial Medical Examining Board. He became president of the Epworth College of Medicine corporation when it was formed in 1907, then professor of ophthalmology, and subsequently head of the otorhinolaryngology department at the University of Oklahoma School of Medicine. Dr. Buxton maintained a large private library; he was a well-educated and brilliant man, a good speaker, and a dynamic leader. His grandson, Dr. Mervin Thomas Buxton, Jr., is now clinical instructor in medicine at the University of Oklahoma School of Medicine. Following Dr. Lauren H. Buxton's death in 1924, the faculty of the University of Oklahoma School of Medicine stated, "The School has lost one of its ablest teachers, a personal friend who exhibited the highest type of loyalty to the school."[7]

Dr. Harry Coulter Todd, M.D., D.Sc., LL.D., was born in Woodstock, New Brunswick, Canada, in 1874. He received his medical degree from Bowdoin College, Maine, in 1900. He came to Oklahoma City in 1902 and four years later became associated, in the practice of medicine, with Dr. Lauren H. Buxton. As one of the founders of the Epworth College of Medicine, and its faculty secretary, Todd delivered the first professional lecture there in 1904. After the Epworth College of Medicine merged with the University of Oklahoma, Dr. Todd became professor of otorhinolaryngology. He was a friendly, refined, highly educated, and philosophical man, with a continuing interest in medical education and an unselfish devotion to true scientific achievement. He was, in addition, an author and poet. Following his death in 1936, an obituary contained this significant sentence, "He and his associates have laid well the foundations of medical education and practice in the state."[8]

Dr. Archa Kelly West was born in Waynesboro, Mississippi, in 1865. He graduated from the Memphis Hospital Medical College in 1894. After practicing at Smithville, Texas, he moved to Oklahoma City in 1899. Dr. West was president of the Oklahoma Territorial Medical Society, from 1904 to 1905. He was an out-

---

[7] *Journal of the Oklahoma State Medical Association,* Vol. XVII (1924), 277.
[8] *Journal of the Oklahoma State Medical Association,* Vol. XXIX (1936), 296.

standing physician, a distinguished speaker, and a truly progressive medical educator. He promoted the establishment and development of the Epworth College of Medicine, and he was its dean during the entire existence of the school.

Dean West was held in high esteem by Oklahoma physicians. He was a leader and a sage adviser, who had many friends and admirers. A memorial resolution by the faculty of the University of Oklahoma School of Medicine on the death, in 1925, of Dr. A. K. West, states:

"A friend of man has fallen. Death has again, with tragic touch, beckoned one of our faculty. The work of Dr. West most surely lives and is not interred with his body. It lives in the School of Medicine which largely owes its existence to his early vision and untiring and unselfish efforts. He leaves a better profession than when he came into the State. He had a hand in the organization of the profession along scientific lines from practically a disordered mob consisting of many good physicians working without concert. He lives and will always live in the hearts of his friends, professional as well as lay. . . . He was calm in adversity, modest in success and capable always."

Dr. Willis Kelly West, prominent orthopedic surgeon and professor of orthopedic surgery at the University of Oklahoma School of Medicine, followed in the footsteps of his pioneering father. Dr. Kelly McGuffin West, of the third generation, is at present professor of continuing education and professor of medicine in the school.

President Evans of the University of Oklahoma had a genuine interest in expanding the School of Medicine and in bringing a proper faculty together. Among the papers of President Evans is a small announcement concerning the School of Medicine of the university. Entitled "Don't Leave Oklahoma to Study Medicine," it explained that a four-year course toward an M.D. degree was being offered and that the School of Medicine of the university had satisfactorily equipped laboratories and clinical facilities and had appointed competent instructors. The June, 1910, university catalog states, "The University of Oklahoma's School of Medicine is now the only medical college in the State of Oklahoma."[9]

The principal change in the faculty consisted in the addition of thirty clinical faculty members, comprising twenty members from the Epworth College of Medicine faculty and ten others recruited in Oklahoma City. There were forty-one faculty members for the year 1909–10 in the Epworth school, and approximately half of the Epworth College of Medicine faculty had volunteered to join the faculty of the University of Oklahoma School of Medicine. The clinical members of the faculty gave their services free of charge to the university, a contribution that continued for many years. They did not receive any compensation other than a very nominal payment, roughly equivalent to the cost of their transportation to and from the teaching hospitals.

By the merger of the Epworth College of Medicine with the University of Oklahoma School of Medicine, some of the most capable physicians in Oklahoma were obtained as teachers and instructors, making it possible for the University of Oklahoma to conduct a four-year medical school. The record of the clinical faculty members who joined the school in 1910 is truly remarkable. Of the thirty clinical faculty members, twelve remained in teaching positions at the university over a period of twenty-five years, and some lived long enough to be appointed to the honor status of emeritus professor. The five who continued longest in the service of the university were the following: Dr. Everett S. Lain, sixty years; Dr. Robert M. Howard, fifty-three years; Dr. Joseph T. Martin, fifty-two years; and Drs. George A. LaMotte and Lea A. Riely, forty-nine years each.

The responsibility of teaching the basic sciences at Norman in 1910 was distributed as follows: Dean Bobo, materia medica, therapeutics, and forensic medicine; Professor Walter L. Capshaw, histology and anatomy; Professor Albert C. Hirshfield, pharmacology and physiology; Professor Henry H. Lane, embryology;

[9] For a list of the faculty of the University of Oklahoma School of Medicine as of June, 1910, see Appendix III.

Professor Louis A. Turley, pathology, neurology, and bacteriology; and Professor Homer C. Washburn, pharmaceutical methods.

Dr. Hirshfield located as a physician in Norman in 1909, prior to his appointment to the faculty as instructor in materia medica in 1910. He then served as professor of physiology in 1911 and 1912, returning to the faculty as instructor in gynecology from 1916 to 1926. Dr. Hirshfield died in Oklahoma City in 1970. Professor Maclaren, whose title had been changed to that of professor of physiology and experimental medicine, resigned as of January 1, 1911, and became professor of physiology at the University of Oregon Medical School in Portland. He retired there in 1934, and died in 1943.

The facilities and arrangements of the School of Medicine in 1910 are described in the quarterly bulletin of the University of Oklahoma general catalog for 1910–11.

"For the present the work in Oklahoma City is carried on at 1005 N. Dewey Street where recitation rooms, laboratories, and libraries are provided. . . . For its clinical work the School of Medicine has the advantage of access to a number of hospitals in Oklahoma City which furnish ample clinical material. The hospitals whose managements have consented most kindly to cooperate with the School of Medicine in this matter are The Oklahoma Hospital for the Insane at Norman [seven hundred beds], St. Anthony Hospital, the Oklahoma City General Hospital, the City Dispensary, the Oklahoma City Maternity Hospital, the Infectious Diseases Hospital, the Smallpox Hospital, the Tuberculosis Hospital, St. Luke's Hospital, and Rolater's Hospital, all in Oklahoma City whose population is over 75,000 persons. . . . St. Anthony Hospital,[10] which has 130 beds, is the largest institution of its kind

10 St. Anthony Hospital, at 601 N.W. Ninth Street, was founded in Oklahoma City in 1898 by the Third Order of the Sisters of St. Francis. Its first building (twenty-five beds) was erected in 1899. It became affiliated with the University of Oklahoma School of Medicine as a teaching hospital in 1910. The Rolater Hospital, at 325 N.E. Fourth Street, was established in 1906, by Joseph Bryan Rolater, M.D. The Central State Hospital at Norman was established in 1895 by the Oklahoma Sanitarium Company. It was later incorporated as the Oklahoma State Hospital. It was opened on June 15, 1895, under Dr. John H. Threadgill. Dr. David Wilson Griffin, a man of character and ability,

in the State of Oklahoma. The Sister Superior has conferred upon the faculty of the School of Medicine of the University the right to nominate three members of the resident's staff for St. Anthony Hospital. . . .

"The new Oklahoma City General Hospital (Third and Stiles Sts.) has 25 beds and an emergency department. The Public Dispensary in the City Hall treats 100 patients daily. The Oklahoma City Maternity Hospital[11] has 12 beds, and many of the patients are treated by the medical students at the patients' homes. The Infectious Diseases Hospital has 10 beds. The Smallpox Hospital has contained one hundred cases at times. The Tuberculosis Hospital has a capacity of 35 beds. All of these city hospitals are in charge of a member of the faculty of the School of Medicine. Faculty and students use this and other clinical material, which averages three hundred patients daily. St. Luke's[12] and Rolater Hospitals are accessible for study to the faculty and students. The Orphan's Home furnishes material for the study of children's diseases.[13]

"The Clinical Library. The clinical library contains a small but well selected list of textbooks and works of reference, and new editions and publications are being added constantly. The reading room is supplied with a sufficient number of leading medical periodicals. The librarian is constantly in attendance to aid workers in their investigations. [Miss Elizabeth Youngman was librarian and clerk. She received an M.D. degree from the School of Medicine in 1911.]

"The University aims to make the School of Medicine thoroughly modern and to offer medical instruction which conforms to the highest approved standards. The hope is that the doctor of

---

came to that hospital in 1899. Later the hospital became affiliated with the University of Oklahoma School of Medicine as a teaching hospital. In 1915 the state purchased the institution and named it Central State Hospital and later Central State-Griffin Memorial Hospital.

11 The Oklahoma City Maternity Hospital was said to have been located on West Main Street.

12 St. Luke's Hospital was apparently a private hospital operated by Dr. Foster Kendrick Camp in 1910 in the Campbell Building, 10 North Broadway.

13 For locations of early medical facilities, see map on page 96.

medicine thus trained will become a trusted leader in his community, a credit to his profession, and a valuable servant of the state.
The medical service which secures the comfort, health, efficiency,
and life of the individual will aid in securing the soundness and
efficiency of the state by love of the work and the best obtainable
education.

"The student of the third or the fourth year must consult with
the local adviser, Professor Archa K. West, M.D., at his office in
the Majestic Building in regard to his work, and receive a statement signed by the local adviser of the classes in which he is to be
enrolled. . . . As the work of the curriculum in professional schools
demands all the time and energy of the student, he should not
attempt to earn any part of his expenses while attending a professional school."

The University of Oklahoma did not acquire any physical facilities, such as classrooms, laboratories, or equipment, from the Epworth College of Medicine. During the year 1910–11, the clinical
faculty, under the leadership of Dr. West and Dr. Buxton, made
informal arrangements for clinical teaching in some of the Oklahoma City hospitals, chiefly Rolater and St. Anthony hospitals.

The additional fees required of students in the Oklahoma City
portion of the medical course were: clinical pathology, $10; hos-
pital, each semester, $20; obstetrics, $10; operative surgery, $10;
and surgical clinics, $10.

Curriculum for Two Years of Clinical Training: 1910

COURSE	THIRD-YEAR HOURS	FOURTH-YEAR HOURS
Clinical Pathology	80	80
Dermatology	64	0
Eye Diseases	32	32
Forensic Medicine	0	32
Genitourinary Diseases	0	32
Gynecology	48	48
Medicine	64	96
Clinical Medicine	256	176
Nervous Diseases	32	48
Ear, Nose, and Throat Diseases	32	32

Obstetrics	64	64
Orthopedics	0	48
Pediatrics	48	48
Surgery	96	192
Clinical Surgery	256	176

The complete curriculum consisted of 37 credit hours in the first year, 34 hours in the second year, and 40 hours in each of the last two years, a total of 151 credit hours or 4,392 clock hours.

The University of Oklahoma School of Medicine was erroneously credited with seven graduates for the year ending 1910 who had actually received their M.D. degrees from the Epworth College of Medicine.[14] Among the group were Dr. Marvin Elroy Stout and Dr. Walter W. Wells, who later became members of the faculty of the University of Oklahoma School of Medicine.

At a meeting of the regents on December 12, 1910, the president of the university reported: "It will be absolutely necessary to make provision for the work of the Medical School in Oklahoma City. In my judgment, it would not be wise yet to enter upon any plan for the permanent group of state hospital and medical school buildings. I would recommend that the Regents authorize me, or appoint a special committee, to see if arrangements cannot be made for the lease of sufficient land in the block where the City Hospital of Oklahoma City is erected, to put up a building with accommodations for class rooms, laboratories, and a state dispensary. . . . I believe that $25,000 would be enough to put up such a building for all present purposes. . . . I recommend further that the Regents should seek authority and means to purchase a suitable site for the Medical School buildings in Oklahoma City. There should be enough land in this for the campus of the Medical School and hospital grounds and . . . some additional close by which might be leased in the future for occupation by benevolent institutions desiring to take advantage of the medical attendance which can be supplied from the State Medical School. . . . Next in order, I believe we must place a medical building here (in Norman) with sufficient ac-

14 *Educational Number of the Journal of the American Medical Association*, Vol. LV (1910), 674; *Bulletin of the University of Oklahoma*, No. 36 (June, 1910).

commodations . . . for anatomy, physiology, and other biological sciences."

At the same meeting a committee was named to decide upon a suitable person to be appointed as dean of the School of Medicine. Members of the committee were Dr. J. Matt Gordon, of Weatherford; Wallace Perry, of Lawton; Robert C. Betty, of Temple; and the president of the university.

Certain conclusions may be drawn about the creation of the four-year School of Medicine at the university, a historic and progressive action undertaken solely by the regents and president of the University of Oklahoma. The state legislature had no part in this timely, judicious decision, so vital to the survival of medical education in Oklahoma. In fact, meager financing by the state and delay in provision for an Oklahoma City campus and buildings proved tremendous handicaps for medical education in Oklahoma during the eight ensuing years and made it inevitable that the acceptable class A rating of the School of Medicine would have to be withdrawn. Only the allegiance and dedication of an enlightened and indefatigable faculty kept the school intact under such trying circumstances.

V.   Today's Opportunism, Tomorrow's Mistake: 1911

THE POLITICAL BACKGROUND was highly complicated in the young state of Oklahoma in 1911. Displeased with the location of the capital at Guthrie, which he termed a "Republican nest," Governor Haskell was instrumental in getting a constitutional amendment, in regard to the location of the capital, presented to the voters on June 11, 1910. When it became clear that the voters preferred Oklahoma City, Governor Haskell declared Oklahoma City, the geographical center of the state, to be the new capital city. Guthrie civic leaders brought suit, but the state supreme court upheld Haskell's action, and on appeal to the United States Supreme Court, it was affirmed in May, 1911, that the voters of a state could determine the location of the capital despite an enabling act restriction.

Lee Cruce, the banker and lawyer from Ardmore who had failed to obtain the Democratic nomination for governor in 1907, ran again in 1910 and won the primary election over William H. Murray. Cruce defeated Joseph W. McNeal, a Republican banker from Guthrie, in the November election, thus becoming the second governor of Oklahoma. Lee Cruce had originally migrated from Kentucky to the Indian Territory and had married Chickie Le Flore, a daughter of a prominent Choctaw family.

Governor Cruce was of a cautious nature. After taking the oath of office at the new Capitol in Oklahoma City, he went to Guthrie and had the ceremony repeated a second time! He initiated an economic program which encountered considerable trouble with legislators. Also, he became the center of bitter political opposition because of his plans to abolish some of the state-supported colleges and to tighten control over others, including the University of Oklahoma, by way of a new State Board of Education.

On January 24, 1911, soon after taking office, Governor Cruce attended a special meeting of the State Board of Regents in Oklahoma City. A president and secretary were elected, but only for a day, as this turned out to be the terminal meeting of the first State Board of Regents. Dr. J. Matt Gordon and President A. Grant Evans were authorized to attend the February meeting of the Association of American Medical Colleges, at the expense of the university. A motion was passed that the board's committee on appropriations ask the legislature to appropriate $75,000, instead of merely $25,000 as recommended at the December 12, 1910, meeting, to secure a site and to erect buildings at the School of Medicine. To do this, the board shifted $75,000 from the amount requested for a building for the Law School.

On March 6, 1911, at the insistence of Governor Cruce, the third legislature created a new central governing board, known as the State Board of Education, and on April 8, the governor appointed the members of this board. This new State Board of Education took over the functions of the former State Regents of the University of Oklahoma.[1] The board promptly ordered a reorganization of the medical school in order to bring it fully abreast of the requirements in medical education at that time. It has been said that Governor Cruce had no direct knowledge of medical education, and some felt that he was dependent on the counsel of Dr. J. C. Mahr, of Shawnee, the state commissioner of health at the time, for advice in this area.

The Council on Medical Education made its third tour of inspection of medical colleges during 1911 and the early part of 1912, visiting only forty-three of the schools for a third time, including the University of Oklahoma School of Medicine. Following this inspection, the School of Medicine of the University of

[1] For a list of the members of the Oklahoma Board of Education, 1911–19, see Gittinger, *The University of Oklahoma*, 212–13.

Oklahoma was declared acceptable in respect to the courses in medical sciences on the Norman campus.

Important administrative changes in the state's educational institutions were taking place at this time. The minutes of the State Board of Education indicate that on April 26, 1911, Dr. Archa K. West appeared before the board and made a statement in regard to the School of Medicine. Two days later the board voted not to renew the appointments of A. Grant Evans as president of the university and the appointments of certain members of the University of Oklahoma faculty, including Dean Bobo of the School of Medicine. Likewise, a number of heads of other state schools were not reinstated.

The board was criticized widely for these actions, especially for its summary dismissal of President Evans. According to Charles F. Long: "The Haskell political machine had caused the University to undergo a disheartening setback. President Evans' one desire was to operate the school on a strong administrative basis and improve scholastic standards, but he was unable to escape from under the wing of Haskell's [governing board], which insisted upon handling most of Evans' administration themselves. As a result, between 1908 and 1912 political meddling in University affairs damaged its reputation, and the scars were visible far beyond the State's boundaries. Many of the faculty, politically appointed, were poorly qualified."[2]

At the May 22 meeting of the State Board of Education, Dean J. C. Monnet was unanimously selected to become the acting president of the university. On May 26, Dr. West again appeared before the board with President Evans, to make statements of concern about the School of Medicine. The board appointed a committee to confer with the new acting president of the university and to recommend someone as a candidate for the position of dean of the medical school. On June 14, the board voted to retain those faculty members of the School of Medicine who were teaching at Norman. At a meeting on June 17, it fixed the salary for the dean

2 Charles F. Long, "With Optimism for the Morrow," *Sooner Magazine*, Vol. XXXVIII (September, 1965), 33.

of the School of Medicine at three thousand dollars a year, and on June 29, the board passed a resolution of policy that all appointments to state institutions should be for an indefinite period. After any person had served two years to the satisfaction of the board, his appointment would be presumed to be permanent.

In the meantime, President Evans made a farewell address to the students of the university in the chapel at Norman on May 31. During his tenure he had seen the School of Law established (1909), the College of Engineering organized (1909), and the expansion of the School of Medicine from a two-year to a four-year program (1910).

At the August 2, 1911, meeting of the State Board of Education, Dr. Robert Findlater Williams, of Richmond, Virginia, was present by invitation and was unanimously elected dean of the School of Medicine to succeed Dean Bobo as of September 1, 1911. During the year the office of the dean was moved from 1005 N. Dewey Street to 317 N.E. Fourth Street in Oklahoma City.

Dr. Williams was born in 1869. He received his M.D. degree from the University of Virginia in 1892, after which he spent a year in research in Vienna. In 1894 he became an instructor in the Medical College of Virginia; in 1895, adjunct professor of histology, pathology, and bacteriology; in 1896, instructor in surgery; in 1897, clinical lecturer in orthopedic surgery; in 1901, professor of materia medica and therapeutics and clinical lecturer in medicine; and in 1904, professor of the theory and practice of medicine. He retired in 1906, moved to El Paso, Texas, and then returned to Virginia to become superintendent of Catawba Sanitorium, prior to his selection as dean of the University of Oklahoma School of Medicine.[3] In 1914, after resigning his position as dean, Dr. Williams returned to Virginia, residing near Charlottesville. He died in 1916.

One week after the election of Dean Williams, the board of education met to hear a report by Dr. Augustus G. Pohlman.[4]

[3] *Virginia Medical Semi-Monthly*, Vol. XXI (1916), 156; Wyndham B. Blanton, *Medicine in Virginia in the Nineteenth Century* (Richmond, Garrett and Massie, 1933).

[4] Dr. Augustus Grote Pohlman was born in 1879. He received his M.D. degree from the University of Buffalo in 1900, and was professor of anatomy at the Indiana Univer-

Dr. Pohlman had, by invitation, previously consulted members of the board on the subject of medical education at the University of Oklahoma School of Medicine. His report, dated August 4, was apparently never made available to the faculty, though it is very significant.

"Advance of the work of the Arts Department at Norman has been checked by sectarian and political intrigue. Her condition is both anomalous and unhealthy. . . . I would have the Board bear in mind the mistakes of its predecessors. . . . It was decided by the State Board of Education, on the advice of interested as well as disinterested practitioners of medicine, that the full four year course in medicine must be continued. . . . I submit this scheme (not materially different from what I proposed in my meeting with the Board)." Dr. Pohlman then made the following suggestions:

"That the four year course be continued, that fifteen units of entrance requirements obtain for the year beginning September, 1911." Dr. Pohlman then discussed details for adapting the basic science courses in the School of Medicine to eliminate the use of the Arts and Science faculty, with the exception of Dr. DeBarr. Following various suggestions concerning individual teachers at Norman, Dr. Pohlman stated: "The equipment in chemistry is . . . the only good equipment in the medical school; that in bacteriology is fair, and the remainder poor. . . . That beginning with 1912 some of the [basic science] departments be moved to Oklahoma City. This idea will be tried here at Indiana University next year. . . . That a premedical course of two years be organized, beginning September, 1911, and that this plus the first two years of medicine entitle the student to a B.S. in Medicine. . . . That the permanent staff of qualified men to take charge of the work of the first two years of medicine be elected in September 1912. [Pohlman stressed a need for those with proper experience and research interest.] . . . . That efforts be made toward securing about $20,000 per year for the medical departments at Norman.

"That the State Board of Medical Examiners be requested to

---

sity School of Medicine in Bloomington, Indiana. He was a member of the American Association of Anatomists and of the American Medical Association.

raise the requirements for entrance upon the study of medicine to two years of collegiate work. This would give time for the proper erection, organization and equipping of a State Hospital at Oklahoma City (a thing which certainly must come). It gives time for the proper selection of a permanent and efficient dean. . . . That the staff of the clinical years at Oklahoma City be reappointed for the year, that a dispensary service be organized, . . . that the clinical pathologist have quarters rented from St. Anthony Hospital; that a nominal fee be paid each instructor per hour; that an acting dean be appointed. Dr. West, because of his experience and attitude toward medical education, is well qualified to take charge of this work. He understands the situation thoroughly. . . . The President of the University should have complete control over the appointment of the dean. . . . That all effort be made at the coming legislature for funds to build and maintain a State University Hospital in Oklahoma City. Also that an effort be made toward an opening of and working relation with the present dormant City Hospital. Oklahoma City has a great possibility as a medical center, probably not surpassed even by New Orleans. There is no large hospital within a radius of 300 to 400 miles. It will take three to five years to get it going. . . . I believe that Dr. Rolater has a very important offer which might work wonders in the establishment of this institution. The City Hospital would be an ideal place to organize a dispensary service.

"Opportunism has brought about a chaotic condition in the University work, and what may seem to be an opportune thing today may be a grave mistake tomorrow."

At that same meeting the board heard the observations and recommendations of Dean Williams regarding the University of Oklahoma School of Medicine, citing such authorities as the Association of American Medical Colleges, the Council on Education of the American Medical Association, and the Carnegie Foundation for the Advancement of Teaching. "The American people," he said, "are suffering by thousands today through the great number of ignorant physicians who have gained diplomas from commercial schools. . . . The Medical School of the Univer-

81

sity of Oklahoma must be a standard institution if it is to reflect credit on the State or even continue in existence."

Williams went on to outline medical school costs. He cited the University of Kansas Medical School in Kansas City as receiving $170,000 from the state for clinical teaching alone and the University of Texas Medical School as receiving $95,000, plus student fees. Tulane Medical School cost $101,000 a year, with the state and city providing more than one half of this amount. Williams recommended a uniform student fee of one hundred dollars a year, after the 1911–12 session, at the University of Oklahoma School of Medicine.

"The estimated cost for the coming year," he continued, "is $16,750, including $6,000 at Norman, $3,000 dean's salary, $3,500 for the Oklahoma City teachers, $1,200 rent for school building, and $400 to establish an outpatient department."[5]

Dr. Williams, at the instruction of the board, recommended the appointment of the faculty of the School of Medicine for the coming year. His recommendations, which were approved by the board, included all of the 1910 faculty members except Drs. Leila Andrews, Walter Bisbee, Charles Bobo, Thomas Burns, Richard Foster, Everett Lain, Joseph Martin, Homer Washburn, Arthur White, and Arthur Will.[6] Nine additional faculty members recommended by the dean were also appointed in 1911. They were John Archer Hatchett, M.D., professor of obstetrics and gynecology; Robert Findlater Williams, M.D., professor of clinical medicine; Robert Lord Hull, M.D., lecturer on eye, ear, nose, and throat diseases; Joseph Brown Rolater, M.D., lecturer on clinical surgery; William Merritt Taylor, M.D., lecturer on children's diseases; Leigh Festus Watson, M.D., lecturer on operative surgery; Edgar Elmer Rice, M.D., instructor in gynecology; Ralph Vernon Smith, M.D., instructor in surgery; and Frank Bruner Sorgatz, M.D., in-

---

5 At the December 12, 1910 meeting of the regents, President Evans recommended a budget for the School of Medicine of $19,000 for 1911–12 and $18,700 for 1912–13. The *Session Laws* and the university catalog for 1911 show appropriations of $171,732 a year for the entire university.

6 The Department of Forensic Medicine came to an end with the termination of Dr. Bobo's faculty appointment.

structor in medicine. Later in the year, six additional members were appointed: John Davidson Rue, M.A., associate professor of chemistry; John Mosby Alford, M.D., instructor in medicine and anesthetist at University Hospital; Joseph Campbell Ambrister, M.D., instructor in genitourinary, skin and venereal diseases; Annette Cowles, R.N., instructor in nursing and superintendent of the University Hospital; Edward Francis Davis, M.D., instructor in ophthalmology, otology, rhinology, and laryngology; and Casriel J. Fishman, M.D., instructor in clinical microscopy. Thomas Bell Winningham was appointed clerk of the School of Medicine and served until 1914.

Dean Williams also recommended demotion in grade for fourteen clinical professors to the rank of lecturers. His reasoning is apparent in the following quotations from his recommendations:

"I find that the work of the scientific years at Norman is acceptable, but that of the clinical years at Oklahoma City is not. . . . The immediately imperative needs lie in the clinical work in Oklahoma City. . . . The existing conditions in the clinical department rob the school of its proper authority in this regard [dependence on clinical material offered by the clinical teachers from their own private practices, etc.]. . . . The clinical teachers in Oklahoma City have given their services . . . without compensation. I recommend payment of a graded scale of fees for hours actually spent. I find that last year there were 18 full professors in the School in Oklahoma City. Such a body is too unwieldy to do efficient work. . . . I therefore recommend the immediate reorganization of the teaching staff in Oklahoma City . . . as follows: 1) Professors, who shall constitute the voting faculty. They shall be heads of departments directly responsible to the dean, their fee to be $3.00 per hour; 2) Lecturers (or demonstrators or directors), responsible to the professor of their department and to the dean, their fee to be $1.50 per hour; 3) Instructors, responsible to the lecturer or professor of the department, with a fee of $1.00 per hour. The necessity with which I am confronted . . . largely deprives me . . . of choice in selection of the faculty, since the clinicians of the city have private control of the facilities and material essential to us. . . . The time [before the beginning of the next semester] will be very short after my return about September 1, 1911."

At its September 29 meeting, the State Board of Education heard further statements by Dean Williams and Acting President J. C. Monnet. The board accepted the plan which had been outlined by Dean Williams for the medical school. A rumor had spread, prior to the board meeting, that a group of the clinical professors at the University of Oklahoma School of Medicine might be demoted to the status of lecturer, or be dismissed, and when the demotions in rank were actually announced, the action was exceedingly disturbing to many clinical faculty members. Many were convinced that Dr. J. C. Mahr, the state commissioner of health and a supporter of Governor Cruce, had advised Dean Williams, on a personal basis, to recommend the dismissals. Furthermore, some felt the failure of the State Board of Education to reappoint ten reputable clinicians who had rendered satisfactory services was, to say the least, a rather heavy-handed way to solve academic problems. In protest, Drs. Abraham L. Blesh, Lauren H. Buxton, and H. Coulter Todd sent their resignations to the board, which accepted them summarily October 3, 1911. It is to the credit of the university that most of these professors were later reinstated without loss of tenure. According to a statement by Dr. Everett S. Lain, the next president of the University of Oklahoma, Dr. Stratton Brooks, in 1912 demanded the restoration of these clinical teachers to the faculty of the School of Medicine with resultant harmony and cooperation in the school.[7]

There were forty-six faculty members in the School of Medicine during the academic year 1911–12, according to the university catalog and Roy Gittinger's *The University of Oklahoma, 1892– 1942*. The names of Drs. Blesh, Buxton, and Todd were included, but only five of the ten not recommended by Dean Williams were listed. The other five were recognized as faculty members in 1912– 13, with unbroken tenure, making a corrected total of fifty-one faculty members for the year 1911–12.

The first recorded meeting of the faculty of the School of Medi-

[7] Everett S. Lain to Mark R. Everett, October 21, 1967.

cine was held in the office of Dr. Archa K. West on September 23, 1911. Those present were Dean Williams and Drs. Edmund S. Ferguson, John A. Hatchett, Robert M. Howard, William J. Jolly, and A. K. West. At this meeting Dr. Ferguson was selected as the first secretary of the faculty of the four-year school. At two subsequent meetings during 1911 a resolution was passed that clinical faculty members be recompensed according to the credit hours of their teaching; it was suggested that a reference library be established in the college building (the rented Rolater Home at Fourth and Stiles Streets); a library committee was appointed, consisting of Drs. George A. LaMotte, Horace Reed, Lea A. Riely, and A. K. West, with an advisory hospital committee (Drs. Robert M. Howard, Joseph B. Rolater, and William M. Taylor); and it was suggested that the professional privileges of the state university hospital be limited to the officially appointed teaching staff.

In 1911 the Oklahoma State Medical Association recommended the establishment of a hospital for the state medical college: "Proceedings of the House of Delegates, Convened in Leighton Building, Muskogee, Oklahoma, May Eleventh, 1911, at Nine A.M.

"Whereas, there exists an imperative need for an institution of state-wide importance for the proper medical treatment of the indigent sick, thus relieving the various counties of a condition many of them are unable to meet, and at the same time affording the most advanced facilities for this work,

"BE IT RESOLVED, that the State Medical Association of Oklahoma hereby endorses the establishment and maintenance of a state institution for the treatment of the indigent sick, an institution to be conducted in connection with the State Medical College."[8]

In an editorial in the *Journal of the Oklahoma State Medical Association*, Dr. Archa K. West endorsed the creation of a state hospital under the jurisdiction of the School of Medicine of the University of Oklahoma (as at the University of Minnesota in 1909). Dr. West stated that the school had been ranked as one of five four-year schools in the South acceptable to the Council on

[8] *Journal of the Oklahoma State Medical Association*, Vol. IV (1911), 34.

Medical Education, and he stressed the need for the new hospital to retain this rank.[9]

Because the temporary arrangements that had been made by the clinical faculty for the year 1910–11 were inadequate, the university had to arrange for rented quarters in Oklahoma City. At the August 9, 1911, meeting of the State Board of Education, Dean Williams said, "I have taken up the question of leasing the City General Hospital with the Commissioners, but their conditions preclude the use of that building. I have also investigated the possibility of utilizing the building of the Epworth University. A suit to foreclose a mortgage of $40,000 on the property has just been instituted and therefore no legal lease is possible."

The board then authorized a committee, consisting of R. H. Wilson, the president of the board; Dean Robert Williams; and a third member, to confer with the city commissioner and the chamber of commerce in regard to a hospital for the School of Medicine. Subsequently, at its September 29 meeting, the board approved a contract with Dr. Joseph Brown Rolater to lease his hospital and home at N.E. Fourth and Stiles Streets in Oklahoma City, as a hospital and quarters for the School of Medicine, for a period of ten years at an annual rental of six thousand dollars.[10] Dr. J. B. Rolater was a physician of considerable energy and personality. He was interested in financial and business affairs, with some concern for medical education.

In an informational article on the reorganization of the School of Medicine, Dean Williams states: "The reorganization of the School of Medicine of the University of Oklahoma was undertaken for the purpose of immediately elevating its standard to the requirements of Class A institutions, as defined by the Council on Medical Education of the American Medical Association and the Association of American Medical Colleges.

"An essential requirement for this standard is that a medical school shall control its own hospital. This condition had not been

9 *Ibid.*, 205.

10 *University of Oklahoma Bulletin*, New Series, No. 112, Biennial Report (July, 1916), 126.

previously possible of attainment by the University Medical School, and to accomplish this end our energies were first directed. Hearing that the city was not in condition to conduct the City General Hospital, which was nearly completed, we made tentative proposals to the commissioner looking to the acquisition of the city's hospital. Our proposition was at first cordially received, but opposition to the plan subsequently developed which led the commissioner to name conditions impossible of acceptance by us, so that our proposition was withdrawn and the plan abandoned.

"While this matter was under consideration, Dr. J. B. Rolater came forward with a generous offer to enlarge his private hospital to meet our needs, and to lease us his hospital and adjacent residence for a term of ten years at a very reasonable annual rental, and this offer was accepted.

"The residence provides us with a beautiful school building which any medical school would be proud to occupy. The handsome exterior attracts immediate attention by its beauty and dignity. The interior is finished throughout in hard wood and has been handsomely equipped, in harmony with the building, with durable and serviceable furniture.

"On the first floor are the general office, the dean's private office, the library and the clinical laboratory; while the second floor contains lecture rooms for the junior and senior classes, a study room and a rest room for students, [also, according to the March, 1912, university catalog, a clinic room for the use of special sections of the classes].

"The additions to the hospital are being pushed rapidly and we expect to get possession of the building early in December. The addition will increase the capacity of the building from 22 to 64 beds. When completed, the hospital will contain 26 ward beds. The wards for white men and white women will have nine beds and those for colored men and colored women four beds each. The rest of the beds will be in private rooms, a few of which will contain two beds.

"In the basement will be located the free dispensary for walking patients, a most valuable adjunct to our teaching facilities. This department will be comfortably arranged, with waiting rooms for white and colored patients, and private rooms for examining patients and instructing students.

"The school opened October 2nd, and is now in full running order, with a faculty and student body enthusiastic in this work. The courses have been arranged, with regard to subjects required and the number of hours given in each, exactly according to the requirements of the Association of American Medical Colleges for the standard of Class A institutions.

"The quick development of such an institution as we have, without special appropriation by the Legislature, has taxed the financial strength of the University, but the Board of Education, recognizing its need, directed that the plan be carried out and the authorities of the University have concurred generously in the furtherance of the development of the Medical School. All of these gentlemen, by this recognition of the claims of the medical profession to the largest consideration in our highest institution of learning, have won the approbation of the profession throughout the state.

"Through the courtesy and interest of the Medical Faculty, a library is being developed by gift and loan of books, and subscription to medical journals, which will do the school infinite credit and be of untold benefits to both faculty and students. In several instances whole libraries have been loaned with the prospect of donation later.

"The State University Hospital (formerly Rolater Hospital) will have as Superintendent Miss A. B. Cowles, a lady of large experience in hospital management, and at present Superintendent of the Colonia Hospital in Mexico City.

"A Training School for nurses will be conducted under the direction of the Superintendent, Miss Cowles. Here in a three-year graded course every facility will be offered the young women of the state for a thorough and rounded training in the art of nursing."[11]

On October 12, 1911, the State Board of Education renamed the rented hospital the State University Hospital, and it reaffirmed

11 *Journal of the Oklahoma State Medical Association*, Vol. IV (1911–12), 302.

the name of the medical school as the University of Oklahoma School of Medicine. At this same meeting Annette B. Cowles was appointed as superintendent of the University Hospital.

The hospital was occupied on January 17, 1912, after it had been remodeled to provide classrooms, executive offices, clinical laboratories, and a dispensary.[12] Thus for the first time the university had under its control the facilities for its clinical teaching.

The clinical laboratories were reported ready on November 11, 1911. The outpatient department was ready on February 1, 1912. The March, 1912, university catalog stated the following in regard to the free dispensary in the basement of the hospital:

"It has separate clinic rooms for the departments of eye, ear, nose, and throat; children's diseases; medical and nervous diseases; genitourinary and skin diseases; and surgery. This dispensary is open daily, except Sundays, from one to three o'clock and the students here do the work under the direction of the dispensary staff, rotating in sections through the whole dispensary service. Each [fourth-year] student here has twenty hours of actual work in each department, except medicine and surgery, in which he has forty hours each. Many clinics are held daily in the hospital, the arrangement being shown in the published schedule."

The catalog also states: "The School building was formerly a beautiful private residence. It is located at 317 N.E. Fourth Street and adjoins the State University Hospital. The library contains some 400 volumes consisting of textbooks, reference books and bound periodicals covering the entire field of medicine, and 15 of the leading current journals are supplied in the reading room." These books and journals, donated principally by members of the faculty, were the nucleus of the School of Medicine's library in Oklahoma City. A separate smaller library had been formed on the Norman Campus in 1911, by transferring a few appropriate books and journals from the general library of the university to a room in Science Hall.

12 The announcement in the *Journal of the Oklahoma State Medical Association*, Vol. IV (1911–12), 393, that the University Hospital (formerly Rolater Hospital) opened on December 17, 1911, is in error.

One of two Oklahoma City hospitals which were connected with the teaching program of the School of Medicine at this time was St. Anthony Hospital, with its 130-bed capacity and a staff composed exclusively of members of the faculty of the School of Medicine. The sisters of St. Anthony Hospital were very graciously accorded teaching privileges in regularly held clinics in that institution.

The Holmes Home of Redeeming Love developed from the Oklahoma Rescue Home for Oklahoma and Indian Territories. Established by the Free Methodist Church of North America in 1900 in Guthrie, it was moved to 5401 Portland Avenue, Oklahoma City, in 1910, as the Holmes Home of Redeeming Love. It was founded by Mrs. Pearl Holmes and Miss Anna L. Witteman. The establishment offered a quiet retreat for obstetrical cases, and it extended teaching privileges to the School of Medicine. Students in small groups were permitted to attend cases with the visiting physicians who were members of the School of Medicine faculty. In 1931 a twenty-four-bed hospital was added, and in 1948 it was incorporated into the present Deaconess Hospital. A maternity dispensary was also established by the School of Medicine at 530 W. Elm Street. A visit to this site (now S.W. Thirteenth Street) revealed that the area had been leveled, probably in connection with improvement of the nearby North Canadian River bed.

Well-equipped pathological and bacteriological laboratories were maintained both in Norman and in Oklahoma City. The laboratory in Oklahoma City was especially equipped, with facilities for making immediate examinations in connection with cases arising in the hospital work. In fact, the 1912 university catalog paints a rather glowing picture of conditions: "Excellent school accommodations were provided and the necessary hospital control acquired so that the School of Medicine, now well equipped with every essential for good teaching, and manned by a carefully selected corps of experienced teachers, offers today a thoroughly modern course of instruction which conforms to the highest approved standards. Applicants for admission to the school are advised to secure one or two years of college training in chemistry, physics and zoology."

A total of 4,407 clock hours of instruction was included in the medical curriculum for the year 1911–12. In the first year the student had 1,232 hours; in the second year, 1,072 hours; in the third year, 923 hours; and in the fourth year, 1,180 hours. "Clinical instruction is given wholly in small sections so that every student has opportunity for personal observation of cases . . . under this arrangement every student received individual instruction from every member of the teaching corps."

The established student fees were $50 for the first year, $30 for the second, $100 for the third, and $105 for the fourth. In June, 1911, fifteen M.D. degrees were conferred. The members of this first graduating class of the four-year school were Walter B. Adams, Herman Gustav Brandes, Walter Traynor Dardis, Elmer E. Darnell, John Wesley Francis, Katherine Josephine Kelly, Samuel Frank LeFevre, James R. McLaughlin, William Ewell Montgomery, J. Arthur Mullins, Leon Lewis Patterson, A. Sylvester Piper, Blair Points, Virgil May Wallace, and Elizabeth Katherine Youngman.[13] There were fifty-three medical students enrolled for the academic year 1911–12.

A brief summary of the complicated events which transpired during 1911 may be helpful to the reader. In an effort to have a central board manage all state-sponsored education, Governor Cruce, during the first year of his administration, prevailed on the third legislature to terminate the State Board of Regents and create a new State Board of Education in its place. It was his hope that this board would eliminate some of the educational institutions in the state and control others in the interest of economy.

The new governing board promptly removed A. Grant Evans, president of the University of Oklahoma, and Dr. Charles Sharp Bobo, dean of the School of Medicine, unwarranted actions which provoked severe criticism in national educational circles.

[13] For subsequent classes, only those graduates who became faculty members of the University of Oklahoma School of Medicine will be named.

Having imported a new dean, Dr. Robert F. Williams, for the medical school, the board veered to the side of propriety by securing advice from a capable nonpolitical consultant on medical education—Dr. Augustus Pohlman. Had the board followed more completely this consultant's forward-looking constructive advice, it might have avoided fulfilling his parting prophecy that "what may seem opportune today may be a grave mistake tomorrow."

Dean Williams, after offering certain progressive recommendations, dismissed some worthy members of the clinical faculty, causing considerable resentment and alienating some of these physicians at a time when their support was sorely needed. On the positive side, Williams did attempt to arrange for the rental of a suitable teaching hospital, only to be badly handicapped by the austere financial provision from the state. A stopgap measure by the State Board of Education was the temporary leasing of the Rolater Hospital until such time as a teaching hospital might be built. This step proved to be not so temporary, and it led to a very precarious situation in regard to the rating for the medical school.

Meanwhile, the first recorded faculty meetings of the School of Medicine were held in 1911, and fifteen graduates received the first M.D. degrees granted by the University of Oklahoma.

VI. The First University Hospital: 1912–14

A GRAPHIC CARTOON, entitled "Why Does It Not Rise?" and depicting the attempted ascension of a balloon labeled "Our Reputation as a University," appeared in the 1912 *Sooner Yearbook*, the university annual. The overweight passenger in the balloon was the "Board of Education," with the word "Politics" on his collar. Charles F. Long brought the picture clearly into focus:

"Every school man in the nation knew that the fledgling University of Oklahoma was the Peck's Bad Boy of the nation's collegiate educational institutions. The East was still in a state of shock since the summary discharge of President Boyd and part of the old Oklahoma faculty by the Haskell regime.

"Mr. Wilson, President of the State Board of Education, said, 'our State Board of Education also controls the normal schools of Oklahoma and has been accused of playing politics in the appointment of the presidents of them. In fact, Governor Cruce has summoned us for trial on that charge and we feel that it is desirable that we appoint a president at the University whom none of us has ever seen.' "[1]

Actually, the new State Board of Education was hampered considerably by not having access to the minutes of the previous State Board of Regents, in spite of the fact that the secretary of the new governing board had, during 1912, sent several formal requests for a copy of those proceedings to the governor, the president and

[1] Long, "With Optimism for the Morrow," *Sooner Magazine*, Vol. XXXVIII (September, 1965), 34.

ex-president of the university, and the secretary of the previous state regents. In session on October 31, 1912, the board passed a resolution stating that the records of the previous regents of the university had not been turned over regardless of repeated demands. A second resolution was passed declaring that "W. E. Rowsey, C. C. Weith and David I. Johnston are claiming the right to act as members of the State Board of Education, under the pretended appointments made by the Governor of the State on April 8, 1911."[2]

During 1912, Governor Cruce replaced several members of the State Board of Education. Those who were ousted tried to retain their places through a court order. The governor finally called a special session of the State Senate in December to uphold his action, but was declined support by the Senate.

At the March 9, 1912, meeting of the State Board of Education, a letter from the secretary of the Council on Medical Education to Dean Williams was introduced. This letter suggested certain improvements required at the School of Medicine in order to raise its standards. The board appointed a committee to investigate the problem and, at its March 28 meeting, naively authorized the expenditure of $450 for the improvements necessary to bring the medical school to a class A rating.

At the March 9 meeting, the State Board of Education also voted to tender Stratton Duluth Brooks, LL.D., of Boston, the position of president of the University of Oklahoma. The board received his acceptance on March 28. According to Charles F. Long:

"He [Brooks] told them that while he was not interested in the presidency at Norman, if the Board were sincere in its professed desire to place the University on a nonpolitical basis, the new president whoever he might be could not do it, unless the board agreed upon and lived up to two basic principles.

" 'First,' he declared, 'all appointments of faculty and other

2 Further complicating the puzzle was the fact that William E. Rowsey, a member and secretary of the State Board of Regents from 1907 to 1911, was elected its president at the terminal meeting on January 24, 1911. Governor Cruce subsequently appointed him to the State Board of Education. He served from 1911 to 1913. The author has located these "lost" minutes.

employees must be made only on recommendation of the president of the University. No member of the board should recommend directly or indirectly any appointee. The board should vote yes or no but should not substitute for an appointee they reject.'

"Years later President Brooks said, 'Whatever was accomplished during my eleven years as president of the University was possible only because the Board of Education had appointed me, and its successors never violated the basic principles set forth in the first conference.' "[3]

President Brooks is also quoted as saying, "Unlike Bostonians, Oklahomans didn't go in for precedent. Nobody in Oklahoma was interested in your ancestry. . . . Broadly comparing Boston and Oklahoma, I should say, that in Boston everybody was against you if you had a new proposal, but in Oklahoma everybody was against you if you didn't listen to their proposal."

In the 1912 *Educational Number of the Journal of the American Medical Association* the four-year School of Medicine of the University of Oklahoma was no longer listed in class A-plus or A, the Council on Medical Education having lowered the rating on June 3, 1912, to B since the university did not own its clinical facilities. The B rating, which indicated need for considerable general improvement, was not changed until March, 1920, after eight years had elapsed.[4]

According to the *Journal of the American Medical Association* for 1912, a hospital for the university School of Medicine had been leased for three years and remodeled and enlarged to a capacity of sixty patients. The 1912–13 catalog of the University of Oklahoma indicates that this was the State University Hospital at 325 N.E. Fourth Street, in Oklahoma City, which, together with the adjoining Medical School Building, at 317 N.E. Fourth Street, had been leased from Dr. Rolater.

Errett R. Newby, secretary to the president of the University of Oklahoma, stated: "A much larger amount of clinical material will

[3] Long, "With Optimism for the Morrow," *Sooner Magazine*, Vol. XXXVIII (September, 1965), 35.
[4] *Journal of the American Medical Association*, Vol. LXXIII (1919), 510.

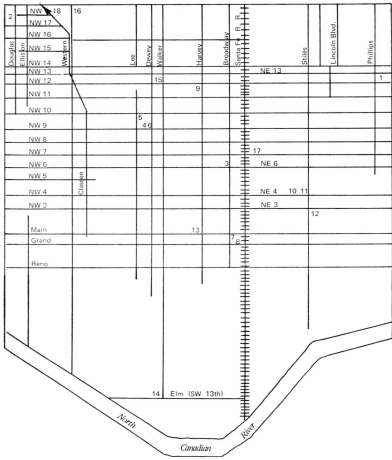

1. University of Oklahoma Hospital (1919) 800 N.E. 13th Street
2. Epworth University College of Medicine (1904) 18th and Douglas Street
3. Epworth College of Medicine (1907) 701 N. Broadway
4. St. Anthony Hospital (1899) 601 N.W. 9th Street
5. O.U. School of Medicine Building (1910) 10th and Lee Streets
6. O.U. School of Medicine Building (1911) 1005 N. Dewey Street
7. St. Luke's Hospital (1910) 10 N. Broadway, 9th floor Campbell Building
8. Wesley Hospital (1911) Herskowitz Building, 11th and 12th floors
9. Wesley Hospital (1912) 300 N.W. 12th Street *(antecedent of Presbyterian Hospital)*
10. Rolater Home (1907) 317 N.E. 4th Street
11. Rolater Hospital (1907) 325 N.E. 4th Street
12. Oklahoma City General Hospital (1911) 400 N.E. 3rd Street (S.W. Postgraduate Hospital)
13. Oklahoma City Maternity Hospital (1910) West Main Street
14. Maternity Hospital (1910) 530 Elm Street
15. Oklahoma City General Hospital (1927) 501 N.W. 12th Street *(antecedent of. Mercy Hospital)*
16. Holmes Home of Redeeming Love (1910) 5400 N. Portland Ave. (4 miles N.W. of 17th and Classen)
17. Oklahoma City Lying—In Hospital (1918) 101 N.E. 7th Street

Locations of medical institutions in Oklahoma City

be available for the third and fourth year students at Oklahoma City than heretofore. There are nearly two hundred beds under the direct charge of the University faculty and our students have access for clinical purposes to other hospitals in the city." The beds referred to evidently included those at St. Anthony Hospital.

From the time Stratton Duluth Brooks became president of the University of Oklahoma, on May 1, 1912, he took a very active interest in improving the School of Medicine. In his August 16, 1912, letter to county commissioners in Oklahoma are the following statements: "In case the present arrangements in your county for taking care of charity cases that need hospital treatment are expensive or unsatisfactory, the arrangements proposed below may be of interest to you.

"The State University Hospital in Oklahoma City will on request of the County Commissioners receive patients and furnish board, lodging, nursing and all necessary drugs and dressings at the rate of $10 per week. No charge will be made for the professional services of physicians and surgeons. Owing to the high standard necessarily maintained at the State University Hospital, the price of $10 per week barely covers the actual cost of the service rendered. The charges for private patients range from $12 to $25 per week.

"Second, to secure clinical material for use in the instructional courses of the university, no case will be demonstrated before students without the consent of the patient.

"Patients will be met at the station with an ambulance when necessary, provided sufficient notice is given of the day and hour of arrival.

"Each patient of course must be properly certified to us by statement, sent in advance or else accompanying the patient, that the county commissioners authorize the reception of the patient by the hospital and that they will be responsible for the charge of $10.00 per week. Each patient should also be provided with a round trip ticket to and from Oklahoma City."

There were five meetings of the faculty of the School of Medicine during 1912. In these meetings it was decided that reputable physi-

97

cians be allowed to admit patients to the University Hospital throughout the summer vacation (June 1–September 15); that one intern from among the 1912 graduates be appointed to the staff of each of the two hospitals—University and St. Anthony—and that each intern receive board, lodging, laundry and five dollars each month; and that Dr. Archa K. West be authorized to pass on credentials of students for admission to the School of Medicine. The minutes report that a full dispensary staff had been appointed by September.

There were fifty-nine faculty members in the School of Medicine in the academic year 1912–13. Fourteen were new appointees. They were Charles Howard Stocking, Ph.C., professor of pharmacy; John Frederick Kuhn, M.D., lecturer on clinical surgery; Curt Otto von Wedel, Jr., M.D., lecturer on minor surgery and bandaging and superintendent of the dispensary; Floyd Jackson Bolend, M.D., instructor in pediatrics; Rex George Bolend, M.D., instructor in dermatology and genitourinary diseases; Howard Storm Browne, M.S., instructor in pharmacy; Isaac Newton Cottle, M.D., instructor in gynecology; Charles Duncan Ferguson, M.D., instructor in eye, ear, nose, and throat diseases; Clarence Henry Field, M.D., instructor in gynecology; William Alonzo Fowler, M.D., instructor in obstetrics; Dolph D. McHenry, M.D., instructor in eye, ear, nose and throat diseases; Earle Sellers Porter, M.A., instructor in chemistry; Andrew Merriman Young, M.D., instructor in obstetrics; and Martha Eggleston Zimmerman, R.N., assistant superintendent of the University Hospital and instructor in nursing. Also appointed were four laboratory assistants: Pleasant Addison Taylor in anatomy and physiology, Herbert Victor Louis Sapper in bacteriology and histology, Harry Slatkin in anatomy, and John Lestrange Rock in physiology.

Clinical departments of the medical school had been organized during the year 1911–12. Two that were listed officially in the 1912–13 catalog were the Departments of Medicine and Surgery. Dr. Archa Kelly West was the first head of the Department of Medicine, which had four subdivisions. These, and their heads, were: pediatrics, Dr. William Merritt Taylor; nervous and mental

98

diseases, Dr. Antonio DeBord Young; genitourinary, skin, and venereal diseases, Dr. Curtis Richard Day; and clinical laboratories, Dr. Casriel J. Fishman. The first head of the Department of Surgery was Dr. William James Jolly. The surgery department's five subdivisions and heads were orthopedics, Dr. Robert Lord Hull; eye, ear, nose, and throat diseases, Dr. Edmund Sheppard Ferguson; gynecology, Dr. Robert Mayburn Howard; obstetrics, Dr. John Archer Hatchett; and radiography, Dr. Everett Samuel Lain. The 1912–13 catalog named Dr. John Smith Hartford as the chief of the dispensary staff. During 1912, Dr. John Mosby Alford taught, under the supervision of the Department of Surgery, the first course in anesthetics to fourth year students, a course which was continued subsequently by Drs. Floyd Bolend and Rex Bolend.

Dr. Gayfree Ellison, who had been appointed in 1910 as instructor in surgical anatomy, became professor of bacteriology and head of the bacteriology and hygiene department established on the Norman campus in 1912. Louis A. Turley's title was thereupon changed to professor of histology and pathology.

Some salaries of faculty members for the year 1912–13 were as follows: Dean Williams, $3,300; Dr. DeBarr, $2,250; Professors Capshaw, Hirshfield, Rue, Turley, and Ellison, $1,500 each; Earle S. Porter, $900; and Dr. Fishman, $50 a month. The total expenditures for the School of Medicine for the fiscal year 1912–13 were $15,950.

Thirty-eight medical students were enrolled for the academic year 1912–13, and ten graduates of the School of Medicine received the M.D. degree in 1912. Each student was required to give six anesthetics, to assist in six obstetrical cases, and to take a total of 4,496 clock hours of instruction. During 1912, the Phi Beta Pi honorary medical fraternity's local chapter was established at the School of Medicine of the University of Oklahoma.

The degree of Bachelor of Science in Medicine, upon completion of the first two years of the medical course, was instituted in the College of Arts and Sciences at Norman, in 1912. In that same year the Training School for Nurses was started on the Oklahoma

City campus. The March, 1913, catalog for the year 1912–13 contains an outline of the three-year course instituted by the new Training School for Nurses at the University Hospital, which led to the diploma of Graduate Nurse. The hospital was registered as a training school by the Oklahoma State Board of Nursing Examiners, and an affiliation was formed with the State Hospital for the Insane at Norman for special training of nursing students. The first faculty of the training school consisted of the medical school faculty members and the superintendent of the University Hospital, the first incumbent being Annette Cowles, R.N., who had the rank of instructor. Her assistant superintendent was Martha Eggleston Zimmerman, R.N., also with the rank of instructor in nursing. High school graduates received preference for admission to the Nurses Training School, and seventeen students were enrolled during the year 1912–13.

In retrospect, it is obvious that 1912 was not a total failure. Governor Cruce finally reacted to mounting public criticism of the State Board of Education by removing several members of the board in 1912. It is true that the governing board was very definitely hampered by the unexplained disappearance of the minutes of the former State Board of Regents for the university, not knowing what steps had been taken officially. Also, there was the embarrassing situation of the class B rating for the School of Medicine, which had been imposed by the Council on Medical Education chiefly because of the lack of an adequate teaching hospital.

However, on the credit side, Dr. Stratton Brooks accepted an appointment as president of the University of Oklahoma after the board agreed to leave all future recommendations concerning faculty members and employees at the university to his discretion. The new and capable president immediately became actively interested in the School of Medicine and its growth. Furthermore, arrangements were made for reimbursement of the University Hospital, by the various counties, for the medical services rendered to their charity patients; the Department of Medicine and the Department of Surgery were organized; and a Training School for Nurses was opened under the direction of Annette Cowles.

The fourth legislature of the state of Oklahoma, angry with the Cruce administration for proposals to liquidate certain colleges, retaliated by launching extensive investigations of several executive departments in 1913. Governor Cruce came very close to being impeached. Indeed, he escaped that fate by a single vote in the investigating committee, in spite of the fact that he was regarded as a man of high integrity by many.

It was of particular interest to the School of Medicine that Dr. Francis Bartow Fite was appointed to the State Board of Education on January 30, 1913. He remained on that board until its termination in 1919. Dr. Fite was also president of the State Board of Medical Examiners from 1912 to 1913, a capacity in which he worked very closely with Dr. LeRoy Long, of McAlester, who was destined to become dean of the School of Medicine at a later date.

On May 14, 1913, the House of Delegates of the Oklahoma State Medical Association passed a resolution complimenting Governor Cruce for his appointment of Dr. Fite, an outstanding physician in the state, to the State Board of Education. It was further resolved that Dr. Fite's advice and opinions be given great consideration as to the needs of the medical department of the university. Copies of this resolution were sent to Governor Cruce; Dr. S. D. Brooks, the president of the university; and to R. H. Wilson, president of the State Board of Education.[5]

The minutes of the State Board of Education for February 28, 1913, include the appointment of Dr. William James Jolly as acting dean of the School of Medicine and professor of surgery, at a salary of $1,500, to succeed Dr. Robert Findlater Williams, who had resigned as of February 1, 1913. Dr. Jolly was born in Marion County, South Carolina, in 1849. He graduated from the Medical College of South Carolina in 1882, and came to Oklahoma in 1890. He was one of the founders of the Epworth College of Medicine, vice-president of the corporation, and a professor of surgery there, a title which he held subsequently in the University of Oklahoma School of Medicine, from 1910 to 1914, when he resigned to devote himself fully to the practice of medicine. He

[5] *Journal of the Oklahoma State Medical Association*, Vol. VI (1913), 38.

was still engaged in private practice at the time of his death in 1940, at age ninety-one.

The 1913 *Educational Number of the Journal of the American Medical Association* reiterated the classification of the University of Oklahoma School of Medicine as one of the twenty-one B schools. Only six of these were members of the Association of American Medical Colleges. Needless to say, this lowered status of the school had become an increasingly troublesome problem for the State Board of Education.

On October 24, 1913, President Brooks reported to the board that he had received an interesting communication on October 22, from Dr. Foster Kendrick Camp. Dr. Camp was then a professor of medicine in the Southwest Postgraduate Medical College and superintendent of the Southwest Postgraduate Hospital. He had had experience in hospital operation prior to organizing and operating the Wesley Hospital, at 300 N.W. Twelfth Street. Wesley Hospital had been opened as a private hospital in 1910, for the care of the patients of Dr. Abraham Blesh and Dr. Horace Reed, who moved to Oklahoma City from Guthrie.[6] In his letter Dr. Camp offered to act as superintendent of the University Hospital (formerly Rolater Hospital) until the termination of the university's lease with Ida Rolater on October 1, 1921. His proposal included closing of the Southwest Postgraduate Hospital at 400 N.E. Third Street (with consent of the city commissioners and the Board of Directors of the Southwest Postgraduate Medical College, which had a lease on the Oklahoma City General Hospital until June 20, 1915); renting the Oklahoma City General Hospital

6 Originally Wesley Hospital was the small St. Luke's Hospital housed in the Campbell Building at 10 N. Broadway. It moved, as Wesley Hospital, in 1911 to the top two floors of the Herskowitz Building at the northeast corner of Grand and Broadway. In 1912, Wesley Hospital moved to a converted apartment house at 300 N.W. Twelfth Street. According to an article in *Harlow's Weekly*, Vol. XXI (August 18, 1922), 10, the Oklahoma City Clinic, organized in 1919, purchased the fifty-bed Wesley Hospital in 1919 from Dr. Foster K. Camp. The original staff of the clinic included Dr. A. L. Blesh, head, and Drs. W. W. Rucks, Sr., M. E. Stout, W. H. Bailey, J. Z. Mraz, and D. D. Paulus. Dr. J. C. MacDonald joined the staff upon the purchase of Wesley Hospital. A new sixty-bed addition to the hospital was built in 1926, and a nurses' home, accommodating fifty to seventy-five nurses, was constructed in 1929. The Wesley Hospital was the predecessor of the present Presbyterian Medical Center.

(presently called the Postgraduate Hospital); and arranging for all clinic patients at the Oklahoma City General Hospital to become university clinical teaching cases. The board appointed a committee to investigate this involved proposition.

A series of professional announcements by the Southwest Post-graduate Medical College,[7] which were also carried in the *Journal of the Oklahoma State Medical Association* for 1912, lend some clarity to the situation. An August announcement provides the information that the college had opened in December, 1911, and that it "has taken over the management of the new City Hospital, which will hereafter be known as the Postgraduate Hospital. . . . All strictly charity cases from any part of the Southwest will receive free medical and surgical treatment, the hospital expenses alone being required."

The June announcement of the Southwest Postgraduate Medical College listed among the college's twenty-three faculty members, the names of fifteen physicians who were also members of the faculty of the University of Oklahoma at one time or another: Drs. L. Haynes Buxton, president, Arthur W. White, secretary, A. L. Blesh, A. A. Will, H. C. Todd, E. S. Lain, J. W. Duke, C. E. Lee, J. F. Kuhn, W. E. Dixon, M. M. Roland, L. E. Andrews, L. M. Westfall, J. T. Martin, and J. M. Finney. In the August to November announcements of the college, seven of the above names no longer appeared on the faculty, but three new ones were added, including Dr. W. J. Wallace (later on the university faculty) together with Foster Kendrick Camp, M.D., superintendent of the Postgraduate Hospital and professor of medicine, who was never on the School of Medicine faculty.[8] In the August, 1912, announcement, Dr. Everett S. Lain was designated as secretary of the Southwest Postgraduate Medical College. According to Dr. Lain, its

[7] The Southwest Postgraduate Medical College, located at 400 N.E. Third Street, in Oklahoma City, was listed as a postgraduate medical college in the 1912 and 1914 editions of the *American Medical Directory*.

[8] It is true that at its January 14, 1914 meeting the State Board of Education voted to appoint Dr. Camp as instructor in theory and practice of nursing, but his appointment was evidently not effected, since it appears in no official record of the university. Dr. Camp was listed as a member of the Oklahoma State Medical Association in 1911, 1912, and again in 1916. He later moved to Altadena, California.

faculty decided to lease the hospital after becoming acquainted with Dean Williams' recommendations of August 9, 1911, to the State Board of Education.

On October 25, 1913, the day following Dr. Brooks' presentation of Dr. Camp's offer, two proposals were submitted in writing to the State Board of Education by the Board of Directors of the Southwest Postgraduate Hospital. They proposed, first, to annul their contract with the city of Oklahoma City and with Dr. F. K. Camp, in regard to the Oklahoma City General Hospital building and the care of the city poor, if the state would get permissive arrangement with said parties; or, second, to turn over to the state medical school the clinics of the Postgraduate Hospital subject to present contracts, the state medical school to have full and free use of all the clinics, subject to supervision by a committee composed of the dean of the Medical School, the president and secretary of the Southwest Postgraduate Medical College, and Drs. A. L. Blesh and Lea A. Riely.

The committee of the State Board of Education recommended that this second proposal be accepted, and that the Southwest Postgraduate Medical College's Board of Directors be tendered an expression of appreciation for their proposal. The committee report was adopted unanimously, and the offer was duly accepted by the State Board of Education about three months later. However, at the February 24, 1914, meeting of the board, President Brooks reported that the Board of Directors of the Southwest Postgraduate Hospital had now withdrawn its offer. The State Board of Education automatically rescinded its former acceptance of the proposal, without comment. It is easy to understand, with all these confusing changes, why frequent incorrect statements appeared in various sources concerning the leasing of Oklahoma City General Hospital by the School of Medicine in 1913. Such statements were unwittingly based on an invalidated agreement.

Meanwhile, it was learned that Dr. F. K. Camp had made yet another offer to President Brooks on December 26, 1913 (prior to the State Board of Education's acceptance on January 14, 1914, of the October 25 proposal). This offer provided for a joint training-school program for nurses between the University Hospital and the Wesley Hospital. The proposal was that the university should lease the top floor of the Southwest Postgraduate Hospital for the training school and that, in return, clinical cases in Wesley Hospital should be made available for medical school teaching purposes and any cases coming to the Postgraduate Hospital should be turned over completely to the School of Medicine.

The anticlimax of all this maneuvering was that only very limited informal arrangements were ever made with the Southwest Postgraduate College for clinical teaching in 1913. The School of Medicine did not gain control of the Oklahoma City General Hospital building, which accommodated the Southwest Postgraduate Medical College, until 1915. Dr. Everett S. Lain told the author in 1967 that the Board of Directors of the Southwest Postgraduate Medical College held on to its lease until it expired in 1915 in order to force the building of a new State University Hospital. It is quite possible that a number of the directors had this in mind, but there may have been some more subtle reasons too.[9]

There were five faculty meetings during the academic year 1913–14. Dean Jolly and President Brooks were present at the February 7 meeting, when a resolution was passed regretting the resignation of Dean Robert F. Williams and commending him for his ability, conscientiousness, and character. The resolution was signed by W. J. Jolly, M.D., acting dean, and E. S. Ferguson, M.D., secretary.[10] A motion was passed that the dean and the senior faculty make a report to the president of the university on a reorganization of faculty titles in the interest of conformity with the custom of the university. The senior faculty met afterwards and recommended that there be five professorial heads of clinical departments, namely, medicine, surgery, obstetrics and gynecology, ophthalmology, and otology, rhinology, and laryngology. The senior faculty, as defined, consisted of the professors and associate

[9] See *Harlow's Weekly*, Saturday, June 21, 1913, concerning the rejection of a request by an officer of the Oklahoma State Medical Asociation that the State Board of Education remove a certain member of the faculty of the School of Medicine.

[10] *Journal of the Oklahoma State Medical Association*, Vol. V (1913), 476.

professors: five heads of clinical departments, four associate professors in medicine, four in surgery, one in obstetrics, and one in genitourinary surgery.

At the May 20 faculty meeting the need for journal subscriptions for the library was considered and a plan was devised for entertaining the medical students of the first two years, studying in Norman, at a day-long clinic and banquet in Oklahoma City. At a June 7 meeting, the library committee reported that seventy dollars had been collected for journal subscriptions. Seventeen days later the faculty responded once more when Dean Jolly asked for financial assistance to keep his stenographer through the summer months. Drs. R. L. Hull, L. J. Moorman, Horace Reed, H. C. Todd, and A. K. West were appointed to the library committee at this June 24 meeting. On September 24, Dean Jolly presided at his last faculty meeting. A separate meeting of the Norman faculty of the School of Medicine was recorded on May 27, 1913.

The 1913–14 university catalog lists fifty-four members on the School of Medicine faculty. The 1913 *Educational Number of the Journal of the American Medical Association* gave only thirty-six, obviously an incomplete report. Three new members who joined the faculty during the year were: Leonard Blain Nice, Ph.D., professor of physiology; Charles Earnest Hamner, M.D., assistant professor of bacteriology; Cyril Ebert Clymer, M.D., instructor in surgery. Dr. John Mosby Alford probably served as hospital anesthetist, from 1911 to 1913, since he taught anesthesia to medical students in 1912, but the additional title of hospital anesthetist was given to Drs. Floyd Jackson Bolend and Rex George Bolend in 1913.

Some salaries for the faculty members during the year were instructor, $900; assistant professor, $1,200; professor, $1,600 and $1,700; superintendent of the hospital, $1,200; assistant superintendent, $720. The total expenditures for the School of Medicine were $16,838. The university catalog for 1913–14 showed the total support to the university for that year amounted to $262,863, of which $35,000 was earmarked for a power plant. The catalog stated that tuition was free in all departments of the

106

university. Consequently, in July, 1913, the fees for medical students in the last two years had to be reduced from $100 and $105, respectively, to a flat rate of $10 a year. This also applied to out-of-state students.

Nine graduates received the M.D. degree in 1913, including Robert H. Riley, and there were ninety-four students enrolled in the School of Medicine in the 1913–14 academic year. The clinical courses were listed under five departments: medicine, Dr. A. K. West, head; surgery, Dr. W. J. Jolly, head, subsequently Dr. John Riley, head; obstetrics-gynecology, Dr. John Hatchett, head; eye, ear, nose, and throat diseases, Dr. Edmund Ferguson, head; genitourinary-skin-venereal diseases, Dr. John Riley, head.

The same university catalog contained the first outline of subjects of instruction in the Training School for Nurses; there were no academic courses given. The school had forty-two students in attendance, and the first diplomas of Graduate Nurse were issued to the six graduates. They were Margaret Nevada Jones, Helen Alice Brown Murphy, Abbie Venice Odell, Cora Etta Phipps, May Belle Powell, and Susan Elizabeth Westmoreland.

In the *Bulletin of the School of Medicine* and the catalog of the University of Oklahoma for June and September, 1913, respectively, only the State University Hospital and St. Anthony Hospital were mentioned as teaching hospitals of the School of Medicine. The June *Bulletin for the School of Medicine* stated that an outpatient obstetrical clinic had been organized with a dispensary station in the south side of Oklahoma City in charge of a competent matron, that the State University Hospital contained twenty-six ward beds and thirty-four private beds, and that students were serving as history clerks and keeping the records on all patients. A free dispensary was located in the basement of the State University Hospital with separate clinic rooms for the departments of eye, ear, nose, and throat; pediatrics; medical and nervous diseases; genitourinary and skin diseases; and surgery.

At the December 15, 1913, meeting of the State Board of Education, the resignation of Acting Dean William James Jolly was accepted. Dr. Curtis Richard Day, who had been professor of genitourinary and venereal diseases since 1910, was appointed dean and professor of pathology, serology and clinical microscopy, effective February 1, 1914, at a salary of $3,000. He enjoyed the privilege of using equipment of the university for private practice and of continuing his association with St. Anthony Hospital.

Dr. Day was born near Warrensburg, Missouri, in 1866. He graduated from the Beaumont Hospital Medical College in St. Louis in 1891. Coming to Oklahoma in 1901, Dr. Day was in general practice at Edmond and then at Oklahoma City in 1906. He had political friends, having been a representative from Oklahoma County in the first state legislature (1907–1908), which framed the laws for the state of Oklahoma. Dr. Day served with the rank of captain at Camp Travis, Fort Sam Houston. He became a lecturer on dermatology at Epworth Medical College from 1907 to 1910, and was then appointed professor of genitourinary and venereal diseases at the School of Medicine. In 1914 he became professor of pathology and clinical microscopy. In 1913, Dr. Day had served as secretary of the Legislative Committee of the Oklahoma State Medical Association. Dr. Day resigned from the faculty in 1915; he died in 1931.

On January 1, 1914, the School of Medicine raised its minimum entrance requirements to one year of college credit and a reading knowledge of a modern language (in addition to English), thereby complying with the Council on Medical Education's requirement for class A medical schools. Six days later the School of Medicine was inspected by the council. The class B schools which were members of the Association of American Medical Colleges, including the University of Oklahoma School of Medicine, had been warned to make necessary improvements to avoid having their rating lowered again by the council.

Dr. Colwell, the secretary of the council, reported to President Brooks on July 31 some deficiencies that were evident at the School of Medicine. These included inadequate space for class sessions, lack of sufficient teaching personnel, very insufficient financial support, handicaps to professors in their research efforts, an inadequate medical library, delayed development of basic science departments together with insufficient equipment for them, and ineffective provision for postmortem examinations. The most serious deficiency was in clinical instruction, the teaching cases being so scarce that regular clinics could not be held. In the outpatient department only eight patients were available daily.[11]

The council recommended that the university provide a teaching hospital averaging two hundred patients daily, to be utilized fully for teaching; an outpatient service with sixty or more patients a day; an adequate maternity service; and hospital facilities for children's diseases. In the words of the report, "The present conditions are so serious that the rating of the school is close to the class C line. It is recommended that plans be drawn for these developments, and a campaign for improvement be begun."

At the March 10 meeting of the State Board of Education, Dr. Fite and Dean Day informed the board of a meeting they had had with personnel of the Council on Medical Education in Chicago and of the council's decision to leave the School of Medicine in a class B status.

In 1914, Professor L. A. Turley made some enlightening comments concerning the serious handicaps of the School of Medicine on the Norman campus:

"The library has to use a stock room for its reading room. The pathology museum room has to serve as an office for the assistant professor of bacteriology. The wooden anatomy building is a fire trap with no toilets, no storage tanks, and very inadequate heating. The professor of bacteriology has a 9 ft. by 12 ft. office which is also used as a store room. There is only a 10 ft. by 12 ft. animal house. Histology and embryology have no space of their own. The head of pathology has his office in a technique room. In one small teaching laboratory we hold courses for 32 medical, 98 pharmacy, 32 pharmacology and 20 arts and science students."

11 A descriptive article in the *Daily Oklahoman* for Sunday, March 15, 1914, entitled "Varsity Hospital Model Institution," pictured the School of Medicine occupying two buildings at N.E. Fourth and Stiles Streets (the Rolater Hospital), with 160 outpatient cases in the month of February, sixty hospital beds, and an affiliation with St. Anthony Hospital.

At the February 24 meeting of the State Board of Education, President Brooks presented a request from Dean Curtis R. Day that the private rooms at the University Hospital be made available to patients of members of the Oklahoma State Medical Association, under rules approved by the dean and the president of the university and with the proviso that all such cases be assigned to members of the teaching staff. This action was approved.

In the files of the dean's office is an unsigned copy of an agreement between the School of Medicine and St. Anthony Hospital drawn up in 1914. The principal items in the agreement are that St. Anthony Hospital would furnish clinical cases to the faculty of the School of Medicine, provided the selection and treatment of the cases were entirely within the jurisdiction of St. Anthony Hospital's authorities and staff, and that medical students would be required to conform to the rules and regulations of St. Anthony Hospital. The clinics were scheduled from 8 to 10 A.M. weekdays, and the School of Medicine was to pay St. Anthony Hospital five dollars a student to reimburse cost. On December 8, 1938, Helen L. Kendall, registrar of the School of Medicine, made a note that this agreement had been in effect for years, except that no fees had been paid.

The 1914–15 university catalog listed fifty-eight faculty members in the School of Medicine. Those who joined the faculty in 1914 were: Richard Gray Soutar, B.A., B.S., professor of physical education; William Jones Wallace, M.D., assistant professor of genitourinary diseases; George Hunter, M.D., instructor in obstetrics; John Arthur Reck, M.D., instructor in gynecology; and Herbert Victor Lewis Sapper, B.A., B.S., instructor in bacteriology. Paul Fesler was appointed clerk in the School of Medicine on October 1, 1914.

No meetings of the entire faculty were recorded in 1914, although Professor W. L. Capshaw acted as secretary for several meetings of the Norman faculty. The total expenditures for the school that year were $18,512. The 1914–15 university catalog gave the support for the entire university for the year as $223,150. The State Board of Education provided a sum of $4,000 in the annual budget for the hourly pay of clinical faculty members at the school.

There were fourteen graduates who received the M.D. degree in 1914, including Dr. Carl T. Steen, and the 1914–15 university catalog listed ninety-five medical students enrolled in the School of Medicine for that academic year. No diplomas of Graduate Nurse were issued in 1914, but the same catalog reported that there were thirty-two students in the Training School for Nurses in 1914–15. The catalog also carried an announcement of a new three-month course for advanced study by graduate nurses.

In reflecting upon the period of the Cruce administration, insofar as medical education is concerned, it might be said that these were years of ineffectual sparring and apprehension in which the School of Medicine failed to keep pace with progressive reforms throughout the nation.

The brief span of the deanships of Dr. Jolly and Dr. Day was marked by maneuvers to synchronize clinical instruction in various Oklahoma City hospitals with the program of the School of Medicine. These attempts met with little success, except for the co-operation of St. Anthony Hospital.

At a time when the School of Medicine reached its lowest classification level, with a class C rating impending, a very propitious event occurred, namely the appointment of Dr. Francis B. Fite as a member of the State Board of Education. Like a knight in armor, he was to champion the cause of medical education under the next governorship and to play a substantial role in the long overdue development of the School of Medicine.

VII. A Vigorous Governor and an Able Dean: 1915–16

ROBERT LEE WILLIAMS was elected as the third governor of Oklahoma in 1914. Born in Alabama, he became a Methodist minister in Texas and then taught school and studied law. He moved to Oklahoma Territory during the Cherokee Outlet opening in 1893, returned temporarily to Alabama, and then moved to Durant, Indian Territory, in 1896. Williams was a delegate to the 1906 Constitutional Convention and a year later was elected chief justice of the state supreme court.

Governor Williams was certainly one of Oklahoma's strongest chief executives. He was an able and assertive administrator, determined to support his beliefs with his actions. His high sense of duty and great political ability were important factors in his control of the legislative assembly. Dr. Fred S. Clinton made this observation: "Oklahoma and its people were very fortunate to have the wise counsel and experienced leadership of Governor Williams. His intelligent interest in and recognition of, the vital need of the preservation of the life and health of the people and their medical education was an invaluable contribution to this state. While he was a stickler for the loftiest ethical standards, he believed in progress, and sought the advance of medical science and art along safe and sane lines."[1]

One can say, without doubt, that Williams was the first governor since the beginning of the Oklahoma Territory who had any

[1] Fred S. Clinton, "University of Oklahoma Medical School Crisis Averted," *Chronicles of Oklahoma*, Vol. XXV (1947), 342.

concept of the purposes of higher education and the aspirations of a university. Having looked into the plight of the School of Medicine, he decided to improve it, and to accomplish his goal, he sought the aid and advice of a respected friend whom he had known in Atoka, Oklahoma, Dr. LeRoy Long, of McAlester.

Fortunately, Governor Williams and President Brooks shared a mutual desire to develop the University of Oklahoma School of Medicine. President Brooks held the confidence of the State Board of Education, which never once tried to control him, so he eventually was able to repair much of the damage to the University that had occurred from 1908 to 1912.

Governor Williams took office when World War I was raging in Europe and when adverse economic conditions prevailed in the state. Consequently, he trimmed institutional appropriations generally, in order to reduce the state's indebtedness. However, during his term of office, the state was able to make provision for the construction of the Capitol Building in Oklahoma City, at a cost of one and a half million dollars, and to purchase the private mental hospital at Norman for one hundred thousand dollars, renaming it the Central State Hospital.

Starting in 1912, considerable pressure had developed to find a new and energetic dean for the University of Oklahoma School of Medicine. By 1915 the number of medical schools in the nation had been reduced to ninety-five; they were classified by the Council on Medical Education as sixty-six in class A, seventeen (including Oklahoma) in class B, and twelve in class C.

It was common knowledge that the school had never been especially well promoted from the Norman campus, so what the School of Medicine most needed was a champion with some political influence and a genuine interest in medical education. Dr. Francis B. Fite, of Muskogee, was just such a man, for he, too, had decided that he had a mission to perform—elevating the School of Medicine to an A rating. Being unusually intelligent, and now a member of the State Board of Education, Dr. Fite was determined that medical education in Oklahoma should no longer suffer from lack of adequate support and competent administration.

113

Dr. Francis Bartow Fite was born in Georgia in 1861. He received his M.D. degree in 1886 from the Southern Medical College (later part of Emory University) and started his practice in Tahlequah, Indian Territory, in that same year. During 1888 and 1889, Dr. Fite pursued postgraduate study in New York City, then returned to the Indian Territory to establish a practice in Muskogee. He was one of the medical examiners of the Cherokee Nation in 1890; president of the Indian Territory Medical Association, 1893–94; a member of the Board of Medical Advisors in 1896; president of the State Board of Medical Examiners in 1912 and 1913; and a member of the State Board of Education from 1913 to 1919. He died in 1938.

The State Board of Education found the class B medical school its most harrowing responsibility. Dr. Fite had discussed the problem with Acting Dean W. J. Jolly two years previously, and had approached his friend of territorial days, Dr. LeRoy Long, in 1913 and again in 1914 about serving as dean of the school. Dr. Long said years later: "In May, 1915 I was again requested to serve [as dean]. This time Dr. John W. Duke of Guthrie, with whom Dr. Fite had been in communication, was spokesman. . . . Appeal was made to my sense of duty to the medical profession. I hesitated . . . and the next day I was elected."[2]

Various comments made by Governor Williams indicate that he had discovered the only hospital facilities available to the School of Medicine were some rented from a surgeon whose private practice interests interfered with proper teaching of medical students and that a number of Oklahomans felt it necessary to study medicine in other states because Oklahoma had only a B class medical school. In discussions with the State Board of Education, its members recommended Dr. LeRoy Long for the position of dean; also Drs. Hatchett, John W. Duke, and Fite had all recommended him.[3]

[2] Hayes, *LeRoy Long, Teacher of Medicine*, 62.

[3] Dr. Fred S. Clinton, a leading physician and surgeon of Tulsa and a former citizen of the Creek Nation, was an additional strong supporter of Dr. Long. He had been president of the Indian Territory Medical Association in 1902 and 1903.

Governor Williams then requested the members of the board to secure the resignation of the incumbent dean, or he was going to veto their appropriation. So it was that on May 27, 1915, the State Board of Education, on motion by Dr. Fite, appointed Dr. LeRoy Long, of McAlester, as dean of the University of Oklahoma School of Medicine, to replace Dean Curtis R. Day, as of September 1, 1915. The board also appointed him professor of surgery, his total salary to be three thousand dollars a year.

Realizing that the tenure of office of a dean might be short, Dr. Long recognized the value of establishing himself in Oklahoma City as a professor of surgery so that, in any event, he would be in a position to do the thing he loved best and for which he was trained. What he never could have foreseen was that he would be serving as dean of the School of Medicine for sixteen years, under three university presidents, namely, Presidents Brooks, Buchanan, and Bizzell. In the beginning, President Brooks felt that the appointment of the new dean had been rather summarily forced upon him, but he readily adjusted to the situation and, in due time, became a warm friend of Dr. Long.

LeRoy Long was born January 1, 1869, in Macklenburg County, North Carolina. He graduated from Louisville Medical College in 1893 and was an instructor there in 1894. In 1895 he started practicing in Atoka, but moved to Caddo several months later. Dr. Long married Martha Downing of the Choctaw Nation in 1896 and began his surgical practice in McAlester in 1904, where he developed into a brilliant, successful surgeon.

Dr. Long was president of the Choctaw Board of Health from 1899 to 1904. He was appointed to this board by Greene McCurtain, the last principal chief of the Choctaw Nation. He was also chairman of the succeeding Medical Board of Indian Territory until 1906. Dr. Long was president of the Indian Territory Medical Association from 1900 to 1901, and in 1899 he had already presented a paper on medical education at a meeting of that association. He was a member of the State Board of Medical Examiners from 1911 to 1915, having been appointed by Governor Lee Cruce. In 1913, Dr. Abraham L. Blesh and Dr. LeRoy Long became charter members of the American College of Surgeons, of which Dr. Blesh was one of the founders in 1912.

Contrary to the belief of some who thought that Dr. Long sought and obtained his appointment as dean through political maneuvering in his own behalf, it was probably the hardest decision he was ever compelled to make.

On the day following Dr. Long's appointment, Governor Williams wrote to him as follows: "I hope to see the Medical School make great growth under your administration, and it will give you a great opportunity. This puts you officially in a titular way at the head of the medical profession of the state. . . ."

It is to be recalled that Governor Cruce was believed to have relied on the advice of Dr. J. C. Mahr, state commissioner of health since statehood, regarding problems of medical education, but when Governor Williams took office, Dr. Mahr had to step down.[4] Commenting editorially, the *Journal of the Oklahoma State Medical Association* said: "Dr. Mahr had the misfortune to be a member of the first State Board of Health and many of the embarrassments of his administration had their incipiency during the regime of that board. . . . On the whole the Health Department has accomplished an enormous amount of work, and among the different charges against the doctor, his enemies have never charged that he was sleeping on the job. . . . The greatest obstacle he encountered was from politicians who wanted to get back at the administration of which he was a part. . . ."[5]

Dr. John W. Duke, of Guthrie, who had had a great deal of experience in the field of neurology in New York and Connecticut institutions before coming to Oklahoma, where he built a reputable institution in Guthrie, accepted the appointment of commissioner of health in December, 1915. The medical profession in general looked on his appointment with favor, aware that he had had considerable legislative experience.

Returning to the new dean, it must be said that the condition of

4 On April 12, 1913, a House of Representatives investigating committee recommended that Dr. J. C. Mahr be removed as state commissioner of health because of improper financial affairs and personal habits.

5 *Journal of the Oklahoma Medical Association,* Vol. VIII (1915), 260.

the School of Medicine was abysmal at the time of Dr. Long's appointment. The state had furnished so little support that everyone on its staff was discouraged; the portion of the school on the Norman campus was housed in temporary quarters; there were no full-time clinical teachers in Oklahoma City; indeed, there was no hospital other than the leased Rolater Hospital, and even there the owner reserved certain rights and privileges; there were no provisions for biochemistry and no x-ray equipment; the apparatus and instruments for examination, treatment, and surgical operations were furnished personally by members of the staff. Faced with this situation, it is no wonder that Dean Long made it clear to the authorities that he could not undertake the task of righting conditions at the School of Medicine without some definite provisions for its development.

At the invitation of the State Board of Education, Governor Williams, President Brooks, and Dr. Long attended its June 14 meeting. Dr. Long outlined the improvements required for restoration of the School of Medicine to a class A status. President Brooks reported that he had received a statement from the secretary of the Council on Medical Education regarding the same needs and he discussed, as a basic necessity, the procurement of essential equipment for the School of Medicine. The board responded by approving a sum of four thousand dollars for that purpose.[6] Governor Williams also discussed the medical school problem, and he subsequently authorized the board of affairs to take steps to equip a chemical laboratory, buy x-ray equipment, and secure additional hospital and clinical facilities. The state built two new operating rooms and established an outpatient department in the basement of the Rolater Hospital, which was still being leased by the university at a rental fee of six thousand dollars a year. The offices, classrooms, and library of the School of Medicine continued to be in the adjoining building, where the kitchen was used for a clinical laboratory.

[6] In 1916, four thousand dollars were appropriated as reimbursement to the university for this expenditure. *Extraordinary Session Laws*, 1916, Senate Bill No. 30, Chapter 12, 13.

At the June 14 meeting the board also heard a report from Sam L. Morely, representing the State Board of Affairs, outlining negotiations to rent the Oklahoma City General Hospital, at Third and Stiles Streets, at the rate of $1,200 a year for the School of Medicine. After this meeting, a contract was made with Oklahoma City for use of the hospital by the School of Medicine, and the school assumed the operation of the free outpatient clinic and the use of twenty-five beds in the emergency department. Subsequently, the Oklahoma City General Hospital was leased and converted to a combination school and hospital building, following the expiration of the lease held by the Southwest Postgraduate Hospital, on June 20, 1915.

One of the first official acts of Dr. Long, as dean-elect, was to address a letter, on August 8, to Dr. N. P. Colwell, secretary of the Council on Medical Education of the American Medical Association, stating exactly what facilities the School of Medicine had and specifically what it lacked. Dr. Long wrote further on August 9 that he would urge that two years of college preparation be required for entrance into the School of Medicine and that the required chemistry course should be given in the medical school, and materia medica should be taught there also. "We have gotten control," he said, "of the City Hospital (formerly known as the City General Hospital and the Southwest Postgraduate Hospital). . . . The large residence which has heretofore been used as the medical school building is being converted into a splendid nurses home and training school. . . . The spirit of cooperation which the members of the faculty are showing is very gratifying to me. Everyone seems to be enthusiastic over the prospects."

Dr. Colwell replied by inviting the dean to come to Chicago for consultation, and, accompanied by Dr. Blesh, Dean Long did so. They were joined in Chicago by Dr. Arthur W. White, a personal friend of Dr. Arthur Dean Bevan and Dr. N. P. Colwell, officials of the council. Dr. Long later said, in reference to this conference with Dr. Colwell, "I made the statement that as long as I was dean of the school, the regulations and ideals of the Council would be carried out, that if any circumstances making that impossible should arise, I would retire."

Dr. Long opened an office in Oklahoma City for the private practice of surgery, but he spent all his forenoons working in the School of Medicine, the dean's office being at that time at 325 N.E. Fourth Street. He threw himself into his administrative work with extraordinary courage. His greatest desire was to obtain an A rating for the medical school by convincing the officials in Chicago that the school was no longer a political football, but, on the contrary, that a vigorous effort was being made to place it on a sound enough basis that standards of an A rating could and would be maintained. He was well aware that there was a world of prejudice to be overcome, even in Oklahoma City, and that he must have the influence and co-operation of the clinicians there. Otherwise, his task would be difficult, in fact impossible.

A few months after his appointment, Dean Long said: "At present we are operating two hospitals, the University Hospital (Rolater) and the University Emergency Hospital (Oklahoma City General Hospital) with an aggregate capacity of 100 beds. In addition we have clinical arrangements with St. Anthony Hospital and with several maternity hospitals. . . . We are in B grade, and we believe we are kept there mainly for the reason that the work of our clinical years is conducted in rented property. We do not believe that the Council on Medical Education looks with favor upon this temporary unsettled situation of the school. . . . We must have a large clinical hospital at Oklahoma City. . . with an arrangement through which the counties of the State shall send the indigent sick and crippled and afflicted to us for treatment."

In a pamphlet issued by the university in 1915, entitled "School of Medicine, University of Oklahoma, Norman—A School of High Standards," we find this summation: "Within the last few months active steps have been taken with a special aim of increasing the efficiency of the Oklahoma City, or clinical, end of the school. . . . Several thousand dollars worth of the most modern equipment has been purchased and installed. One of the most important advances has been the acquisition of the City Hospital at Okla-

119

homa City. This is a fine new building [built at a cost of approximately $60,000] at Third and Stiles Streets. It has four floors. . . . The building is now being remodeled in such a way as to utilize the two lower floors for teaching purposes only. The entire lower floor will be used for outdoor dispensary work."

The first mention in a university catalog of this "Medical School Building," on Stiles Street, was in March, 1916, when it was described as follows:

"On the ground floor are the main operating room, a smaller operating room, and a number of examining rooms. On this floor are located the departments which take care of outdoor dispensary, there being from forty to fifty outpatients daily. Students of the senior class are assigned to the different departments and assist in the treatment of patients. On the second floor are the lecture rooms, the main clinical laboratory, the x-ray plant, the library, and a museum. On this floor also are located the dean's office and the office of the clerk of the school. The upper floors are devoted to hospital work, all the patients in this building being used for clinical [teaching] purposes."

According to a notation made by Miss Helen L. Kendall, registrar of the School of Medicine, on December 9, 1938, the Oklahoma City General Hospital was used to house the clinical years of the School of Medicine, until August 1, 1928; some of the outpatient clinics remained in it even until the fall of 1929.

The 1915 pamphlet on the School of Medicine stated that the University Hospital at 325 N.E. Fourth Street would continue to operate, and that the adjoining building at 317 N.E. Fourth Street was being converted to a home for nurses taking training in hospitals under the control of the medical school administration.[7] Mention was also made that the School of Medicine would continue its teaching at St. Anthony Hospital [then 130 beds] and its weekly medical and surgical clinic at the Oklahoma Hospital for the Insane at Norman [seven hundred patients]. There was no

7 The Rolater Hospital and Home were used by the School of Medicine until the state was released from its contract after the new State University Hospital was occupied in 1919.

tuition fee for residents of Oklahoma; the rate of tuition for non-resident medical students depended upon the state from which they came.

Dean Day presided at only one faculty meeting in 1915. In a letter to Dean-elect Long, July 3, 1915, a committee of the faculty requested that he support a pledge by faculty members not to practice division of professional fees under penalty of severance from the faculty. Dr. Long became dean on September 1, and presided at the next faculty meeting on September 7, when textbooks were selected for the library. At a September 27 meeting, President Brooks presided, with Dean Long present. Dr. Hartford reported that a total of 2,692 dispensary patients had been seen during the year. A motion was passed requesting the State Board of Education to institute a requirement of two years of college education prior to entrance into the School of Medicine, effective January 1, 1917, and this prerequisite was authorized at the December 16 meeting of the board. At the December 26 faculty meeting a resolution was passed in memory of Dr. Walter Capshaw who had been professor of anatomy in the School of Medicine at Norman for seven years. Dr. Gayfree Ellison was elected to replace Dr. Capshaw as secretary of the Norman branch of the faculty.

In 1915–16 there were fifty-six members on the faculty, including six new members: LeRoy Long, M.D., professor of surgery; John Williams Duke, M.D., professor of nervous and mental diseases; Winfield Eugene Dixon, M.D., assistant professor of otorhinolaryngology; John Paine Torrey, M.D., instructor in anatomy and physiology; Lucy Rennette Hill (Rennette B. Hill), R.N., superintendent of the University Hospital and instructor in nursing; and Stephen Harry Graham, M.D., assistant in anatomy.

On September 28, 1915, the State Board of Education appointed Dr. Louis A. Turley as assistant dean of the School of Medicine, at a salary of nineteen hundred dollars. Dr. Turley held this appointment until 1928, and again from 1935 to 1939.[8] At the same

---

[8] These are the official dates. In personal notes and reports made by Dr. Turley in 1938 and 1940, he cited his earlier appointment erroneously as "Acting Assistant Dean 1908 (or 1909) to 1920, and Assistant Dean 1920 to 1928."

meeting of the board, tuition was set at twenty dollars a year for the first two years and fifty dollars a year for the last two years of the School of Medicine. Total expenditures for the School of Medicine in 1915–16 were $18,307. The 1915–16 university catalog showed support for the university was $249,500, together with $100,000 for a science building.

The March, 1916, catalog listed eighty-six students in the School of Medicine during the academic year 1915–16. There were twenty graduates who received M.D. degrees in 1915, including Drs. James Jackson Gable, Robert B. Gibson, Stephen Harry Graham, Harry Slatkin, and Willis Kelly West.

The March, 1915 and 1916 catalogs carried the following statement: "The University has control of the clinics at the Holmes Home of Redeeming Love, the Nazarene Home, and the City Lying-In Hospital. These hospitals furnish 150 obstetrical cases a year which are used for clinical purposes by the University." In the 1915–16 catalog a notice appears that the nonresident student was required to pay tuition (at the same rate an Oklahoma resident would be charged by the corresponding state university).

There were fifty-one students in the Training School for Nurses in 1915–16, and three diplomas of Registered Nurse were issued in 1915. During the year Lucy Rennette Hill, R.N., followed Annette Cowles as head of the school for a period of approximately six and one-half months.

Five years had come and gone since the now defunct State Board of Regents of the University of Oklahoma had created a four-year School of Medicine, five years of struggling and fumbling in which governors and governing boards of the university had shown merely a token interest in the plight of medical education in Oklahoma. This stalemate was terminated when a vigorous new leader appeared on the scene in the person of Robert Lee Williams, who was elected the third governor of Oklahoma.

Governor Williams was bent on correcting some of the impediments to the growth and development of the new state. He was especially concerned with the low national rating of the medical school, which reflected adversely on Oklahoma. Together with

122

Dr. Francis Fite, then a member of the governing board of the university, and other influential physicians, Governor Williams was instrumental in prevailing upon Dr. LeRoy Long to accept the deanship of the School of Medicine, an action which turned out to be one of the landmarks in the history of the school, and indeed of Oklahoma Medicine itself, for the new dean commanded the leadership which had been so tragically needed.

Dean Long forged ahead toward the achievement of two main goals, the construction of a university hospital and the concomitant restoration of the class A rating to the School of Medicine, two objectives which were to be realized within the next five years. Thus the new administration began to operate at a very critical turning point involving the continuance or abandonment of the University of Oklahoma School of Medicine.

Dean LeRoy Long took up the gauntlet for the School of Medicine with the Governor of the State of Oklahoma standing squarely behind him. He faced the future with faith, vigor, and vision, as is evidenced by his clarion call to the faculty and the profession: "Men are on the faculty for but one purpose," he said, "to render acceptable service. As we see it, this is a basic essential for an enthusiastic and able corps of teachers that make up, to a great extent, for lack of equipment and other facilities.

"In addition to the full time men at Norman, we have here at Oklahoma City, some fifty active members of the faculty, and there is a perfectly satisfactory esprit de corps. . . . Since our connection with the school, we have been gratified by this unselfish spirit of cooperation.

"We are in B grade, and we believe we are kept there mainly for the reason that the work of our clinical years is conducted in rented property. We do not believe that the Council on Medical Education looks with favor upon this temporary, unsettled situation of the school . . . an unfortunate crippling situation for a department of the University of the great state of Oklahoma.

"If Oklahoma University is to have a medical department of the kind she should have . . . a medical department of real merit, and

123

withal a source of greatest good for the people of the state, we must have a large clinical hospital in Oklahoma City. Our ideal is a 300 bed hospital with an arrangement by which the counties of the state shall send the injured, crippled, sick, and afflicted to us for treatment.

"If each of you will wake up to the opportunity, we will build here the greatest institution of its kind in the Southwest . . . an institution which will be, in the years to come, a monument to the unselfish enterprise of our citizenship and the righteous cooperation of our profession."[9]

Clinical facilities were truly inadequate and quite fragmented, but arrangements were made, nevertheless, to care for sick and needy persons from over the state at University Hospital for the nominal fee of ten dollars a week. There was no extra charge for operating room, anesthetic, or laboratory work. The only requirement for entrance to the hospital was a letter from a physician, or other responsible person, stating that the patient was unable to pay for the service of a physician or surgeon. Furthermore, if an ambulance was needed upon arrival at the railroad station, the hospital furnished that accommodation, too.

Dean Long reviewed the year's work, since his appointment, at a faculty meeting on June 5, at which President Brooks presided. He stressed once more the insufficiency of the clinical facilities and the urgent need to construct a campus-based university hospital, in order to eliminate the present arrangement of a private hospital service controlled by a non-faculty physician (Dr. Rolater). He further stated that Dr. Means, chairman of the Executive Committee of the Association of American Medical Colleges, had deferred an inspection of the school until the fall of the year.

President Brooks reported to the State Board of Education, meeting on August 24, 1916, that Governor Williams had authorized a deficiency allocation of $13,500 for the University of Oklahoma School of Medicine. To say that this was a timely boost for the school would be a great understatement! The total support for the University of Oklahoma for the year 1916–17 was only

9 *Journal of the Oklahoma State Medical Association*, Vol. IX (1916), 295.

124

$300,431. It is easy to imagine that Stratton D. Brooks, as president of the university, looked askance at the apparent power being mobilized for the School of Medicine. On October 23, 1916, he addressed a letter to Dean Long in which he stated that he had not been aware that the school was a member of the Association of American Medical Colleges, and that he did not see any special advantage in it. Nevertheless, he went on to suggest that Dean Long invite Dr. Colwell to inspect the School of Medicine at his convenience, even though, for his own part, he did not believe it was possible to get a fair inspection report from Dr. Colwell.

Governor Williams attended a meeting of the State Board of Education in November, when it met to hear the report of a legislative committee on appropriations. Speaking before the Board, the governor reiterated that the stumbling block which was preventing the medical school from receiving a class A rank was the simple fact that the University Hospital was located in rented quarters in Oklahoma City, with insufficient equipment and laboratory facilities. Faced with this dilemma, he stated that he was recommending that an appropriation of $200,000 be made for a state hospital to be located on state land in Oklahoma City, on the condition that the Emergency Hospital, in Oklahoma City, be donated to the state.

Meanwhile, Dean Long had invited Dr. Colwell to reinspect the School of Medicine and there had been the usual request for more detailed information from Dr. Colwell. On November 29, 1916, Dean Long gave the average daily attendance in the dispensary as thirty patients, with Dr. Wann Langston director of the dispensary laboratory work. The minimum of maternity cases in charge of each student who graduated in 1916 had been six. Students had also gained experience in maternity cases in the outpatient departments of several hospitals, at University and Emergency Hospitals and Bethany Home, under Associate Professor Looney; at City Maternity Hospital, under Instructor Hunter; and at Holmes Home of Redeeming Love, under Instructor Wells.

Dean Long informed Dr. Colwell that the Governor had gone on record, within the last ten days, as being in favor of a capital

125

appropriation of $200,000 of the School of Medicine and that there was a strong probability that Oklahoma City would also donate the city hospital and grounds to the school. He closed this letter by saying: "The longer I work at this job, the more I realize we have many things to do, but we are coming along and I wish you would come down here to look us over. I know you will criticize us, and I believe we need it."

Obviously, this was not the last word in the lengthy exchange of letters, for we find Dean Long, on December 26, listing the average number of patients available for teaching in various hospitals as follows: St. Anthony Hospital, fifty-five to sixty; Wesley Hospital, thirty-five to forty; University Hospital, thirty to thirty-five; and Emergency Hospital, twenty to thirty. All of the patients in the Emergency Hospital were charity patients, as were an average of six out of the total number at the University Hospital. While the medical school also had the use of twenty-five beds at St. Anthony, there was no way of ascertaining an exact figure on the number who were charity patients. The teaching at Wesley Hospital was limited to a clinic given by Dr. Blesh.

Dean Long then stated that the legislature would be meeting in January, 1917, and that Governor Williams would recommend the appropriation of $200,000, which he had favored earlier, for building a hospital to be operated in connection with the School of Medicine. Dr. Long realized that this was a most crucial time in the history of the medical school and that whatever the coming legislature did would have repercussions far into the future. He suggested that the school had already made considerable progress since Dr. Colwell's last visit but that it might be best to defer any reinspection until the legislature had acted upon the proposed appropriation.

An abstract from the minutes of the Tulsa County Medical Society indicates that Tulsa physicians were supporters of Governor William's proposed legislation and that they went on record December 18, 1916, as favoring an appropriation of $200,000 for the establishment of a hospital for the University of Oklahoma Medical School. Furthermore, the society voted to hold a meeting on January 27, 1917, for the purpose of meeting with their legislators. This strong support, in behalf of the University of Oklahoma's proposed hospital, was spearheaded by Dr. Clinton of Tulsa.

Dean LeRoy Long wrote to Dr. Clinton on December 26: "This is a crucial time in our history for I verily believe that not only the present standing, but the future of the School of Medicine, will depend upon what the coming legislature does in connection with it. We have the active support of Governor Williams, the Superintendent of Public Instruction, and other state officials." He wrote in closing: "President Brooks of the University is interested in building up this department. We need your assistance, and I am depending on you."

President Brooks presided at a December 19 faculty meeting at which both he and Dean Long devoted considerable time to pleas for faculty and student participation in a campaign to secure the appropriation to build a teaching hospital for the School of Medicine. A steering committee, appointed for this purpose, consisted of Dr. West, chairman, and Drs. Blesh, Buxton, Ferguson, and Howard.

Throughout these months, when forces were being marshaled for support of the School of Medicine's own hospital, there were smaller steps forward, too. At a faculty meeting on September 25, the medical school library and the outpatient clinic of the University Hospital came under consideration. Rules pertaining to the library were established by the library committee, and it was announced that Duke Vincent, a medical student, was appointed a part-time librarian, at a salary of ten dollars a month. A total of 5,889 patients were reported to have received medical care under the jurisdiction of the medical school in 1915–16 (820 patients at University Hospital, 779 in the clinics, and 4,290 in the outpatient clinic). Dean Long reported to the faculty about the $13,500 deficiency allocation which had been authorized by Governor Williams earlier, in co-operation with President Brooks; and that an animal house had been constructed, at the rented Oklahoma City quarters of the medical school at Third and Stiles Streets, in addition to enlargement of the laboratory and library areas.

127

Twelve of the sixty-four faculty members of the School of Medicine in 1916–17 were newly appointed. They were: Reuben Morgan Hargrove, M.D., professor of anatomy; David Wilson Griffin, M.D., associate professor of mental diseases and medical jurisprudence; Albert Clifford Hirshfield, M.D., instructor in gynecology (returning to the faculty); Edna Holland, G.N., superintendent of nurses and instructor in nursing; Wann Langston, M.D., instructor in pathology and clinical microscopy;[10] George Davidson McLean, M.D., instructor in surgery; Marion Mansfield Roland, M.D., instructor in dermatology, electrotherapy, and radiography; Floyd Melville Sackett, M.D., instructor in gynecology; Fenton Mercer Sanger, M.D., instructor in gynecology; Marvin Elroy Stout, M.D., instructor in surgery; Charles Benjamin Tayler, M.D., instructor in genitourinary diseases and syphilology; and Walter William Wells, M.D., instructor in obstetrics.

Lucy Rennette Hill, superintendent of the University Hospital, with the rank of instructor in nursing, resigned her position on March 15, 1916. She had been succeeded by H. Mary Workman, R.N., who came from the Naval Hospital at Mare Island, California. Miss Workman was appointed April 15, 1916, but her tenure was short because of an unsatisfactory working relationship with Dr. J. B. Rolater. A letter dated July 17, 1916, to Dr. Rolater, with a copy to the Dean of the School of Medicine, was sent by Miss Workman to complain about the conduct of Dr. Rolater towards her as superintendent of the hospital. On August 24, she resigned, having served about four months.

In a July 7, 1916, letter to President Brooks, and in subsequent correspondence, Dean Long explained that Miss Edna Holland, a former member of the State Examining Board of Nurses, did not want to undertake the business cares which devolve upon a hospital superintendent, but was willing to be the superintendent of nurses and to direct the Training School. Her appointment terminated the custom of combining the positions and was a step toward develop-

10 Dr. Langston originally had been appointed as instructor in histology and bacteriology at a salary of one thousand dollars a year, on April 26. His title was changed to instructor in pathology and clinical microscopy on September 1, 1916.

ing the profession of nursing. In consequence, Paul H. Fesler was made chief clerk of the School of Medicine and acting superintendent of the University Hospital, positions which he held until 1927.

Concerning the departments of the School of Medicine, opthalmology and otorhinolaryngology became separate departments in 1916, with Dr. Edmund S. Ferguson and Dr. Lauren H. Buxton as respective heads. These two subjects were listed separately in the 1916–17 general catalog of the university, as were dermatology, electrotherapy, and radiography (Dr. Everett S. Lain, head), genitourinary diseases and syphilology (Dr. William J. Wallace, head), gynecology (Dr. John S. Hartford, head), mental diseases and medical jurisprudence (Dr. John W. Duke, head), neurology (Dr. Antonio D. Young, head), and obstetrics (Dr. John A. Hatchett, head).[11] A fulltime pathologist and an expert anesthetist were on salary in 1916, in connection with the needs of the two hospitals.

In regard to the 1916 curriculum for the School of Medicine, several courses in chemistry were eliminated so that physiological chemistry (later termed biochemistry) was the only chemistry course retained in the curriculum. A separate course in human parasitology was added, as noted in the minutes of a meeting of the Norman branch of the faculty on December 11, 1916. DeBarr Hall, a new chemistry building on the Norman campus, was completed in 1916 and was used, together with the 1904 Science Hall, as quarters for the instruction of medical students.

The 1916 *Educational Number of the Journal of the American Medical Association* reported the following fees for the University of Oklahoma medical students: first year, $55; second year, $43; and each of the last two years, $25. Twenty graduates received the M.D. degree in 1916. Included in this graduating class were Drs.

---

[11] A 1916 letter from Dean Long stating that Dr. A. W. White was to have direction of the Department of Clinical Medicine did not mean that Dr. White was head of the Department of Medicine. In a letter sent to President Brooks on January 14, 1918, Dean Long stated that Dr. Lain had been in sole charge of dermatology, electrotherapy, and radiography "since our reorganization in 1916," and that no one on the faculty had been more active, systematic, and conscientious than he.

Merle Quest Howard, Wann Langston, Richard Clyde Lowry, Thomas Claude Lowry, Pleasant Addison Taylor, and L. R. Wilhite. In 1916–17 there were eighty-five medical students in the school. One Graduate Nurse diploma was issued in 1916, and there were thirty-one students in the Training School for Nurses.

VIII.   The New University Hospital: 1917–19

ON JANUARY 2, 1917, Dr. Colwell, of the Council on Medical Education, notified Dean Long that an inspection would be made of the University of Oklahoma School of Medicine for the Association of American Medical Colleges. Thus began 1917, a year which proved to be most decisive in the history of the School of Medicine, for it was in 1917 that the sixth Oklahoma legislature insured the school's future by providing for a branch campus and for the University Hospital in Oklahoma City.

The act authorizing construction of a hospital and buildings for the Medical Department of the University of Oklahoma was House Bill No. 366 of the Session Laws of 1917. It designated the site of the hospital building, appropriated $200,000,[1] and declared an emergency. The tract of land designated in the bill to become the site of the medical department of the University of Oklahoma was a 15.64-acre portion of the Capitol lands.[2]

Both the appropriation for and the location of the medical department were made on the condition that Oklahoma City grant and convey to the state of Oklahoma, for a consideration of one hundred dollars, the building known then as the Emergency or Municipal Hospital (previously the Oklahoma City General Hospital or the Southwest Postgraduate Hospital), together with its equipment, incidentals, and tract of land located at Third and

[1] In 1919 this amount was increased by $76,000.

[2] This act was cited by Judge Thomas H. Owen in 1931 as evidence that the University Hospital was not independent, but was created as a part of the School of Medicine.

131

Stiles Streets, to become a part of the plant and equipment of the medical department of the State University.

In section three of the act it was provided that any resident of the state could become a patient in the University Hospital by paying such sum a week as the hospital management might charge for room and board. There was to be no charge for medical attendance, treatment rendered, or drugs or medicines administered.

In section four there was the stipulation that the appropriation would become available when the State Board of Public Affairs certified that Oklahoma City had granted and conveyed its Emergency or Municipal Hospital to the state for one hundred dollars or when it had executed a lease to the state of the hospital and site for ninety-nine years at an annual consideration of five dollars.

Section five stated that if Oklahoma City failed or refused to do this, the State Board of Public Affairs was authorized to locate the medical department of the University of Oklahoma in any first-class city in the state of Oklahoma upon such city conveying lands, properties, securities, and monies at the value of $100,000.

Further rules concerning the hospital were given in section six. Authorized as patients were sick, indigent children or residents of Oklahoma, and obstetrical patients—all to be recommended by the county boards of health—also emergency cases and students from the university or other state schools. A certain number of paid beds for private patients was authorized.

The dean of the medical school was empowered to make further rules and regulations to be approved by the State Board of Education or its successors. The use of the hospital was not to be prohibited to any licensed physician or surgeon, and patients were to have the privilege to call any registered physician or surgeon to treat them.

The senate committee at first refused to report favorably on this bill, thus this legislative measure almost failed. In fact, the senate committee to which it was referred recommended that it "do not pass."

Certain physicians in Oklahoma City, among them Dr. J. B. Rolater, were not in favor of the act. Dr. Rolater's opposition, as conveyed to Dr. Fite, was due to his concern about the lease of his hospital; he would stop lobbying against the bill if the lease was not terminated. As previously stated, Dr. J. B. Rolater was interested in financial and business affairs, with some concern for medical education. His reputed opposition to the bill providing for a new University Hospital would seem to indicate that, in the balance, he was actually more interested in financial affairs than in medical education.

Some members of the medical profession came to the assistance of Dean Long and, as stated by Dr. A. C. Scott in 1949, "through the influence of Governor Williams and Senate friends, a movement for reconsideration was made and a meeting of the committee called, to be held in the Senate Chamber. On account of public interest, and particularly of Dr. Long's reputation as a speaker, a large proportion of the Senate and the entire faculty and student body were present. Impassioned pleas by Dean Long and other members of the faculty were made, with the result that the hostile attitude of the Committee was completely reversed."

On February 21, 1917, Dean Long telegraphed Dr. Fred S. Clinton, of Tulsa, and others to wire their congressmen and senators, urging them to support the hospital bill. Thirty years later Dr. Clinton recalled these events:

"Citizens with understanding and civic pride," he wrote, "joined in aiding the Governor and Dean in gaining fundamental financing. . . . the Tulsa County Medical Society was first in the state to endorse the $200,000 appropriation. . . . there was some strong and very influential opposition in Oklahoma City. . . . if the University Medical School's friends and promoters had been less alert, less resourceful, true, influential, firm, or lacking in common horse-trading sense, ignominious, unhappy, depressing failure would have postponed indefinitely the development of the medical school.

"The pioneering work done by Governor Williams, Dr. Fite, Dean Long, and Paul Fesler, with all of those cooperating in securing the needed buildings, equipment, facilities, . . . was a monumental and memorable achievement. . . . This has inspired and

133

formed the firm foundation upon which their successors are able to erect additional large or suitable buildings, an efficient organiza- tion . . . a double service to humanity and the state."[3]

The bill was approved on March 21, 1917, after passage by an overwhelming majority. According to Dr. Hayes, the influence of Governor Williams was a powerful factor in the passage of the bill. After the senate had voted "do not pass," the governor threat- ened to veto college appropriations in general, unless the bill was passed within three days.[4] At a later date, the governor himself said that organized medicine had not backed the bill actively but that he and Dr. Long had been able to achieve its approval and passage.[5]

In 1922, *Harlow's Weekly* carried an interesting discussion of the University Hospital. After mention of the fact that the Emer- gency Hospital was still in use and not yet discarded, the following statement was made: "The Oklahoma School of Medicine owes more to Dr. Long than the ethics and ideals he has given to it; he literally wrung the new University Hospital from the protesting members of the . . . Legislature. When it became known . . . that Dr. Long would address the committee in the Senate Chamber, a large number of senators attended the meeting which was held during the noon hour. Dr. Long convinced his hearers of the necessity for a hospital building, and though his bill continued to have opposition, it was finally passed by a good majority. He did not give up his fight for it, . . . until the last vote had been cast, and it was safe."[6]

There was also a special article by Dean LeRoy Long in the

3 Clinton, "University of Oklahoma Medical School Crisis Averted," *Chronicles of Oklahoma*, Vol. XXV (1947), 342.

4 Governor Williams actually did veto the Capitol dome proposed by the architects for that building. Governor Williams' sister remembered that "the Governor said it would be possible to build a University of Oklahoma Hospital for what the dome would cost. The young state needed a hospital, he figured, worse than it needed a dome for people to look at." See Ed Montgomery's article in the *Sunday Oklahoman*, November 16, 1969.

5 The dean's correspondence indicates that one of the active senate friends was the Hon. S. L. Johnson, of Okmulgee, because Dean Long thanked him for "successful management of the measure. All of us in the School of Medicine are very grateful to you. I wish to thank you, too, for the beautiful tribute to the medical profession."

6 *Harlow's Weekly*, Vol. XXI (March 3, 1922), 11.

Journal of the Oklahoma State Medical Association in which he recounted the support received. "The struggle against bitter opposition to secure that appropriation may not be generally known," he wrote, "but it was waged incessantly until the victory was won. The multitude of friends that rendered unselfish service in the interest of the school at that time cannot be enumerated here. . . . Among them were state officials including members of the Legislature. . . . above all, there was a great army of physicians who were familiar with our needs and who had confidence in our plans and purposes. . . . This multitude of Oklahoma citizens . . . stood like a wall; they not only stood, but they fought. University Hospital was the first result; an A grade medical school was the next result. This successful fight was the crucial period in the history of the School of Medicine."[7]

The 1916–17 general catalog of the University of Oklahoma estimated that the new hospital would have two hundred beds. The subsequent catalog, published in March, 1918, stated that the university, on July 1, 1917, had acquired the Oklahoma City Emergency Hospital[8] building at Third and Stiles streets under a ninety-nine-year lease. This building housed the following medical school quarters: offices, laboratories, classrooms, dispensary, library, and museum. Adjoining the building was the recently constructed animal house and a facility for experimental surgery. From a communication to Dr. Colwell in 1920, we learn also that in 1918, Dr. J. W. Duke, then commissioner of health, was permitted to build a laboratory in the attic of this building and that the only clinical work of the School of Medicine being performed at the Emergency Hospital was in the outpatient clinics. The 1917–18 catalog of the University of Oklahoma stated that there were forty to fifty outpatients daily in these clinics, and the 1918–19 catalog reported seventy-five to one hundred such patients daily. The residence at 317 N.E. Fourth Street was used as a nurses' home.

A copy of an ordinance, dated June, 1917, by the Board of Commissioners of Oklahoma City, authorizing the above lease to

[7] *Journal of the Oklahoma State Medical Association,* Vol. XVI (1923), 289.
[8] So termed by Dean Long in a January, 1918 letter.

the state of Oklahoma, is in the dean's office files. The authorization was for a period of ninety-nine years, at an annual rental of five dollars. The ordinance also authorized the sale of the hospital's equipment for one dollar and empowered the city to contract with the state for the medical care of patients of the city for a period not to exceed twenty-five years from the date of contract. The mayor and city clerk were authorized and directed to execute the proper instruments.

During 1917 and 1918 the School of Medicine took part in the national military effort for the First World War. On April 22, 1917, Dean Long called a meeting of the faculty of the School of Medicine to announce that the surgeon general of the Army had advised that faculty members should apply through the dean for commissions in the reserve and also to consider whether instruction should continue during the summer to assist the war effort. The extension was approved by the faculty.[9] Arrangements were soon made to train medical officers in orthopedic surgery, and a unit of the Medical Reserve Corps, with forty members, was organized among the medical students.

At a joint meeting of the faculty and the student body on April 23, passage of the bill providing for a State University Hospital was discussed by Dean Long.

A third meeting of the faculty was held on May 31, when the granting of M.D. degrees to the graduating class was recommended.

Dr. Turley reported that the sanitarium at Norman would now supply the anatomy department with cadavers, making it no longer necessary to purchase bodies from undertakers. Dean Long mentioned that the Department of Clinical Pathology was starting a program of research work and, addressing himself to the faculty,

---

[9] The United States Armed Forces were well pleased with this venture and wished to continue their relationships with the University of Oklahoma School of Medicine. In the dean's office files is a letter dated November 28, 1922, from the surgeon general of the United States Army, stating that the secretary of war had authorized at the School of Medicine, General Hospital No. 56, and that Major LeRoy Long, Medical ORC, had been assigned as commanding officer. Dr. Long was then promoted to the rank of lieutenant colonel. A letter of December, 1922, listed twenty-seven faculty members and officials of the school in this hospital unit.

he said, "Whatever I have done; whatever I may do in connection with the school has been done and will be done . . . without any purpose except the advancement of the institution to the point where it will be of the greatest service to the people of the state." The faculty then placed a resolution in its minutes in appreciation of the very able services rendered by Dean Long. "His gentlemanly courtesy to members of the faculty has resulted not alone in warm feelings of regard for the Dean, but harmonious relations between members of the faculty."

There were sixty-six members of the faculty of the School of Medicine in the year 1917–18. New appointees during 1917 were Thomas Boyd, instructor in bacteriology;[10] Arthur Brown Chase, M.D., instructor in therapeutics; Austin Lee Guthrie, M.D., instructor in otology, rhinology, and laryngology; Leslie Marshall Westfall, M.D., instructor in ophthalmology; Charles Lincoln White, D.D.S., clinical consultant in dental surgery; and Earl LeRoy Yeakel, instructor in bacteriology. Dr. Cyril Ebert Clymer was appointed chief of the dispensary staff, a position which he retained for seven years. Paul Fesler was advanced in rank to chief clerk of the School of Medicine in 1917. Military leave was granted to Drs. A. L. Blesh, F. J. Bolend, Rex Bolend, R. M. Howard, George Hunter, G. D. McLean, M. Roland, F. M. Sanger, F. B. Sorgatz, and E. L. Yeakel.

Some salaries during that year were: Mr. Fesler, $1,400; Dr. Hargrove, $200 a month from July to August; Dr. Thomas Boyd, $100 a month; and $6,000 total for the visiting clinical faculty, the hourly rates being $1.50 for instructors, $2.00 for assistant professors, and $2.50 for associate professors and professors. The university catalog for 1917–18 showed $413,520 for the support of the university and $200,000 for the new hospital building.

The student fees in the School of Medicine were: first year, $43, second year, $23, and each of the last two years, $25. Twenty-four graduates of the School of Medicine received M.D. degrees in 1917, and four nursing graduates were granted G.N. certificates.

[10] Not recorded in Gittinger's *The University of Oklahoma* but in the State Board of Education minutes.

Among those graduating from the School of Medicine were James Garfield Binkley, Thomas Madison Boyd, Charles Arthur Brake, and Francis Asbury DeMand. There were seventy-five medical students enrolled during the academic year 1917–18 and thirty-six students in the Training School for Nurses.

According to Gaston Litton, "Almost two years passed after Dr. Long's appointment as Dean, before the Legislature provided the support." However, in all fairness, it should be pointed out that two years was the minimum time in which the state could have moved legally toward building a university hospital once the need became urgent. Dr. Long had become dean in September, 1915, after the fifth legislature adjourned. The succeeding sixth legislature opened in January, 1917, and House Bill No. 366 was passed at that session, representing the earliest possible response to Dean Long's plea for support.

During 1918, the Council on Medical Education advanced the requirement for admission to class A medical colleges by including two years of preliminary college work. The council reported fifty-six member schools of the Association of American Medical Colleges in class A and three in class B. In discussing the ratings the council stated that the University of Oklahoma School of Medicine was striving to become worthy of a higher rating, that it had acquired a new campus in Oklahoma City on which was being erected a state hospital, and that the clinical material of the hospital would be entirely under the control of the medical school.

Entrance requirements for admission to the School of Medicine were increased in 1917 to include the two years of college work, comprising one year of biology, one of physics, one and one-half of chemistry, and a reading knowledge of a foreign language.

During May, 1918, Dean Long filled out a questionnaire for Dr. Colwell, in anticipation of an oncoming inspection. The Central State Hospital (formerly the Oklahoma Hospital for the Insane) had increased its bed capacity from seven hundred to eleven hundred; a weekly medical and surgical teaching clinic was continued there.

There were three meetings of the faculty of the School of Medicine during the year. At the June 1 meeting President Brooks presided. He stated that the university was going to try to establish a two-year course in nursing for college graduates. President Brooks presided again at the June 19 meeting. Dean Long reported encouragingly on his recent visit to Chicago, saying that Dr. Colwell thought the council was well pleased with reports about the school and that there would be no question in regard to the outcome of the impending inspection. The dean presided at the third faculty meeting on September 16. There was discussion once more of the relation of the school to the war effort.

There were sixty-six members of the faculty during the year 1918–19, and the university catalog carried the private office addresses for the clinical members of the faculty. Those appointed for the first time were Felix Thomas Gastineau, M.D., instructor in clinical pathology and microscopy; Arthur Rimmer Lewis, M.D., special lecturer on applied therapeutics; and Mary Virginia Sawyer, B.A., assistant in bacteriology. Dr. William A. Fowler was advanced in rank to associate professor of obstetrics, and Dr. John P. Torrey became acting professor of anatomy for the year. Teaching of medical school courses by the Department of Biology was terminated in 1918. The annual salary for Paul Hill Fesler, clerk of the School of Medicine, who was made superintendent of the University Hospital on July 22, 1918, was $1,600, and that for Edna Holland, superintendent of nurses, was $1,200. The university catalog for 1918–19 showed $404,616 for the support of the university and $200,000 for the University Hospital building.

A second series of military leaves of absence was granted to the following faculty physicians: Dr. J. M. Alford, Dr. E. F. Davis, Dr. Gayfree Ellison, Dr. A. L. Guthrie, Dr. R. M. Hargrove, Dr. R. L. Hull, Dr. Wann Langston, Dr. Horace Reed, Dr. L. A. Riely, Dr. F. M. Sackett, Dr. W. W. Wells, and Dr. A. W. White. In 1918, Dr. Frank Bruner Sorgatz, captain in the Medical Corps and assistant professor of clinical pathology, died in service.

Thirteen graduates received the M.D. degree in 1918. Among them were Ray Morton Balyeat, Felix Thomas Gastineau, and

Walter Howard Miles. There were seventy-eight medical students during the academic year 1918–19. Fees for medical students by classes were $58, $40, $20, and $20. Seven graduates of the School of Nursing received the diploma of graduate nurse, and there were forty-three nursing students during the year. The 1918–19 university catalog outlined the three-year course of study for the nurses training program, listed under proper academic headings. In a letter to President Brooks on November 24, 1918, Dean Long made progressive recommendations about the Training School for Nurses, the nursing staff, and new quarters for the nursing students. He also recommended an expert superintendent and well-trained dietitian for the new University Hospital.

The year 1918–19 was the last in Governor Robert L. Williams' term of office. While Dean Long has received justified recognition from many sources as a leader in the events that transpired in relation to the School of Medicine, the key role of Governor Williams has not received sufficient consideration. Throughout the four years that he was governor, he lent the powerful support of his office to the efforts of Drs. Long, Fite, Clinton, and others and to the endeavors of such a tireless nonprofessional man as Paul Fesler. Without this top-level support it is quite possible that the impressive achievement for medical education in Oklahoma during the term of Governor Williams would never have occurred. Ex-governor Williams continued his keen interest in the School of Medicine and the University Hospital long after his term ended. In November, 1919, he wrote to the chairman of the new board of regents of the university urging construction of a nurses' residence and the landscaping of the grounds and mentioning the need for a teaching Department of Dentistry.

James Brooks A. Robertson, of Chandler, who had the active support of Governor Williams, was elected the fourth governor of the state of Oklahoma in 1918 by defeating William H. Murray. Born in Iowa, Robertson came to Oklahoma Territory in 1893, studied law, and was admitted to the bar in 1898. He was the first

140

governor of the state chosen from the area of old Oklahoma Territory.

The seventh state legislature, under Governor Robertson, created a new and separate board of regents for the University of Oklahoma. This, the fourth governing body for the university since its beginning in 1892, remains in charge of the university today. Governor Robertson appointed its first members as of April 9, 1919. Emil R. Kraettli, who was then secretary to the president of the University of Oklahoma, was appointed the secretary of this board, a position which he retained until 1968.[11]

In 1919 the Council on Medical Education and the Association of American Medical Colleges commenced joint surveys of the various schools of medicine throughout the country. As early as February of that year Dean LeRoy Long had written to Dr. Fred C. Zapffe, the secretary of the Association of American Medical Colleges, and to Dr. N. P. Colwell, secretary of the Council on Medical Education, setting forth the improved situation at the University of Oklahoma School of Medicine and expressing the institution's desire to be advanced to class A. He enumerated such improvements as the provision of a campus and construction of a new hospital. He outlined the current request to the legislature for funds to equip the hospital and for sixty thousand dollars to build a home for nurses, also for a maintenance fund to maintain the hospital. Nevertheless, Dean Long was hesitant about the readiness for advancement to class A despite the efficiency of the teaching force. This was because of uncertainty about what the legislature might do.[12] In the meantime, prices had advanced and, due to the war, some delay in the construction of the University Hospital had ensued.

[11] For a list of the regents from 1919 to 1942, see Gittinger, *The University of Oklahoma*, 251.

[12] According to the 1920–21 university catalog, the support for the University Hospital for 1919–20 was $51,060 for salaries, $22,000 for maintenance, and $56,930 for buildings and permanent improvements. Some salaries had improved. For example, the chief clerk of the hospital and the superintendent of nurses both received $2,000 a year; the hospital dietitian, $1,200; supervising nurses, $975; residents, $600; and interns, $300. The support for the remainder of the university amounted to $560,349.

Dr. Robert Lord Hull, associate professor of orthopedic surgery and a major in the Medical Corps, died in service on January 14, 1919. On February 20, Dean Long wrote to Lt. Wann Langston at Base Hospital 108 in France: "We are all broken up over the deaths of Dr. Sorgatz and Dr. Hull. At this moment the hospital situation is 'up in the air' on account of erratic positions taken by some of the members of the Legislature, which is now in session. The building itself is about completed, and it is a splendid building, but we need a good deal more money to put on some of the finishing touches and to buy equipment. I hardly know how the thing will go, but we feel rather hopeful that progressive medicine is influential enough in the Legislature to head off any foolish efforts to handicap the School of Medicine which is so near the goal for which we have been striving for the last three years.

"It goes without saying that we want you back here in the school just as soon as you can get back, provided the Legislature does not destroy it so that there will be no school. If this goes as we hope, you will have many more and much better opportunities to carry on your laboratory work than when you were here before, but I do not believe that you can do any better work because all of us connected with the school felt that your work, when you were here, was A 1 in every particular."

During several months following the armistice some other faculty members, including Dr. Gayfree Ellison, returned to the School of Medicine. It is on record that Dr. Langston returned from France by July 11.

The rented Rolater Hospital[13] continued to be used to some degree after August 1, 1919, when the first patients were admitted to the new 57,000-square-foot University Hospital. Paul H. Fesler was the first superintendent; he was appointed to the position in July, 1918.

On July 22, 1919, Dean Long wrote to President Brooks that it

13 In a report made in May, 1918, Paul Fesler gave the following information concerning Rolater Hospital: capacity, eighty beds; two interns in 1918–19, plus two student interns; no residents; outpatient dispensary open one hour daily for charity patients; charges at the hospital, $2.50 a day. Fees were: operating room, $5.00 and $7.50; laboratory, $3.00; anesthetist, $5.00; and x-ray, $5.00.

was important to determine what to do about the Rolater Hospital. He suggested to the president that he take the matter up with the board of affairs in order to get a satisfactory adjustment. It will be recalled that this hospital had been rented in 1911 for a period of ten years. The termination of the lease on the Rolater Hospital was secured by President Brooks some time after occupancy of the new University Hospital, but the exact date of the transaction was not known, according to Dr. L. A. Turley in a January 12, 1939, memo to Dean Patterson. It is evident that the use of the Rolater Hospital, at 325 N.E. Fourth Street, and the adjacent Home at 317 N.E. Fourth Street, was terminated after the transfer of facilities to the "Medical School Building" (the Emergency Hospital) at 400 N.E. Third Street, which subsequently housed the administrative offices of the School of Medicine, part of the library, and the outpatient department. It was probably because of the latter function that the regents appointed a last superintendent "for the Rolater Hospital," Mrs. W. A. Dersch, on November 1, 1919.

The minutes of the regents for their March 8, 1920, meeting show that a committee representing the War Mothers appeared and requested that "the Rolater Hospital, now operated by the University" be turned over to the War Mothers to be used as a hospital for disabled soldiers. The *Daily Oklahoman* for March 24, 1920, carried the news item: "Hospital Opening Waits on Governor," in which it was reported that a board representing the War Mothers and the American Legion wished to open a state hospital for wounded and disabled soldiers, sailors, and marines in the Rolater Hospital building.

At a special session the legislature appropriated twenty thousand dollars as a first step toward taking over the hospital, with a view to devoting its resources entirely to the treatment of disabled soldiers and sailors.[14] The acting assistant surgeon general of the United States Public Health Service visited Oklahoma in May to investigate the possibility of establishing a service hospital for the care of sick and injured discharged soldiers.[15] The December, 1920

[14] *Journal of the Oklahoma State Medical Association,* Vol. XIII (1920), 153.
[15] *Ibid.,* 231.

issue of the *Journal of the Oklahoma State Medical Association* carried an editorial advocating the building of a hospital for that purpose and decrying what it termed "short-sighted opposition to the plan."

At a November 5, 1921, meeting of the regents the president of the university presented a communication from the Oklahoma City Chamber of Commerce with reference to the location of a Soldiers' Relief Hospital. Dean Long was invited to be present and to discuss the matter.

The 1919–20 catalog of the University of Oklahoma gave the address of the new University Hospital as 800 N.E. Thirteenth Street in Oklahoma City. It stated that the fireproof hospital had just been completed at a cost of approximately $300,000 ($76,000 of which had been appropriated by the seventh legislature to finish and equip the hospital). Its capacity was given as 176 beds, with 25 being in private rooms. Two hundred beds were available in emergencies. The new hospital contained five large sun porches and eight wards, including separate ones for men, women, whites, and Negroes. There were diet kitchens, five operating rooms, laboratories for diagnostic purposes, and modern equipment. A wing of one floor had been set aside for teaching and research laboratories.

Dr. Long wrote Dean Lyon of the medical school at the University of Minnesota: "Patients are received by the hospital in the three ways that you point out. The first class of cases are charity cases, so far as patients are concerned. Such patients are not able to pay anything, and the per diem is paid by the Board of County Commissioners of the county from which the patient comes, by the municipality from which he comes, and so on. The second class of patients pay the per diem themselves, but receive professional service at the hands of our staff without any cost. In this class the hospital requires that the patients bring with them a recommendation from a physician or some responsible citizen setting forth the inability of the patient to pay for professional service. The third class is composed of private patients, and they pay both the hospital and the physician attending them."

The new University Hospital was formally dedicated on November 13, 1919, at 2:00 P.M. in the House of Representatives Chamber at the State Capitol. On the program were Governor J. B. A. Robertson; Samuel W. Hayes, president of the university regents; Dr. Stratton D. Brooks, president of the university; Dean LeRoy Long; Dr. A. R. Lewis, commissioner of health; and Dr. L. J. Moorman, president of the Oklahoma State Medical Association. The dedication was followed in the evening by a banquet at the Lee-Huckins Hotel.[16]

The new University Hospital became a charter member of the Oklahoma State Hospital Association in 1919. The first president of that association was Dr. Fred S. Clinton, and its executive secretary was Paul H. Fesler.[17]

With the new hospital came the beginning of residencies at the University of Oklahoma School of Medicine. Dr. Raymond Lester Murdoch was appointed as the first resident surgeon in 1919.[18] The following year there were a resident in surgery and gynecology and one in medicine and obstetrics.[19] Georgia Helen McDonald was appointed the first dietitian for the new hospital on August 14, 1919. She served until December 1 of that year and was followed by Catherine Goff, who remained for a period of two months.

There were two meetings of the faculty during 1919. At a February 5 meeting Dean Long stated that the cost of a patient's care at University Hospital was about fourteen dollars a week. Due to dereliction in completion of case records, the faculty voted to deny the use of the hospital to the delinquent faculty members until their records should be completed. At an April 9 meeting,

---

16 *Journal of the Oklahoma State Medical Association*, Vol. XII (1919), 335.

17 Fred S. Clinton, "The Beginnings of the Oklahoma State Hospital Association," *Chronicles of Oklahoma*, Vol. XXII (1944), 338.

18 Dr. Murdoch told the author that a succession of physicians returning from the armed services assisted in the resident's duties for short periods during 1919–20. A letter from Dean Long to Dr. Murdoch in July, 1920, indicates that Dr. Murdoch had been the only formal appointee who completed a year of residency (1919–20). "Now that your period of service as Resident Surgeon has just terminated, I am writing to express to you cordial thanks . . . for the great interest you have taken. . . . During the last half of the year, you have had the responsibility of all the departments on your shoulders."

19 Dr. Edward N. Smith, "History of Department of Obstetrics," MS, January 25, 1941.

where President Brooks presided, Dean Long announced that about twenty-five faculty members had seen service in World War I.

In the academic year 1919–20 there were sixty-two faculty members in the School of Medicine. Those appointed during 1919 were David Byars Ray Johnson, M.A., dean and professor of pharmacy; Joseph Clark Stephenson, Ph.D., professor of anatomy; Edward Pennington Allen, M.D., instructor in medicine; Willis Kelly West, M.D., instructor in surgery; Julia Elizabeth Steele, B.A., B.S., assistant in histology and pathology; Mary Ard Mackenzie, G.N., superintendent of nurses (to succeed Miss Holland); and Candice Monfort, G.N., superintendent of nurses (to succeed Miss Mackenzie, who served only three months).

When Edna Holland retired in early 1919, the University Hospital board extended cordial thanks and grateful appreciation from the board and from all the departments of the hospital for her untiring activity in the interest of the Training School. The citation read as follows:

"During the term of her service Miss Holland has had to meet, in the first place, the numerous unusual duties incident to the war, and, in the second place, the peculiarly trying situation in connection with the prevalence of influenza. She met both situations with that poise and energy which is characteristic of her work.

"We believe that Miss Holland deserves special commendation for her service in connection with the influenza situation which she handled successfully with an inadequate but wonderfully loyal and efficient nursing force. On account of these things the Board tenders to her its everlasting thanks."

The fees for medical students of the four classes in 1919–20 were $61, $40, $23, and $23. Anesthesia was still taught by Dr. Floyd Bolend under the Department of Surgery. An effective maternity clinic had been organized at the new University Hospital; the faculty also supervised the clinics at the Holmes Home of Redeeming Love and the outpatient work which had been developed in patients' homes.

146

In 1919, twelve graduates of the School of Medicine, including Wencelaus T. Andreskowski, received their M.D. degrees, and eight nursing graduates were awarded G.N. certificates. During the 1919–20 academic year there were in attendance eighty-six medical students and thirty-four nursing students. The nurses' home remained in the Rolater Building at 317 N.E. Fourth Street until 1919.

In September, 1919, the university established a student health service at the Norman campus with Dr. Gayfree Ellison, professor of bacteriology, in charge.

It is important to reaffirm the decisive nature of the events during this period. The creation in Oklahoma City of a branch campus of the University of Oklahoma to provide for its future medical center and the construction of a University Hospital specifically designated by the legislature as a teaching hospital for the School of Medicine were of the greatest importance. Authority for the operation of the University Hospital was placed definitely with the governing board of the university and the dean of the School of Medicine. The Oklahoma City General (or Emergency) Hospital was also acquired by the university under a longterm lease to provide an outpatient facility. The medical profession in the state of Oklahoma recognized the importance of these accomplishments, and it co-operated with the university in securing the campus and the building.

During 1917 and 1918 faculty members of the School of Medicine assisted actively in the national military effort of the First World War. Two of these physicians, Drs. Hull and Sorgatz, died in active military service; the others began to return in 1919. At this juncture there was agitation for a state hospital for veterans. Use of the Rolater Hospital, which was no longer essential to the university, was proposed for this purpose by interested civic groups and the newly organized American Legion.

The present Board of Regents of the University of Oklahoma was created in 1919. During the year Dean Long was in communication with the officials of the Association of American Medical

147

Colleges and the Council on Medical Education, looking toward re-accreditation of the School of Medicine in recognition of the considerable improvements that had been made. The University Hospital was dedicated in November, 1919, and its first resident surgeon was appointed that year.

IX.   The Class A Rating Restored: 1920–22

THE YEAR 1920 is a year to remember in the annals of the School of Medicine, for that was the year in which the school was elevated to its former status "in the galaxy of worthwhile medical schools." On January 16, 1920, Dr. Colwell wrote Dean Long that he and Dr. William Pepper of the University of Pennsylvania would inspect the University of Oklahoma School of Medicine on January 30. Following the inspection, Dean Long informed Dr. Colwell, on February 16, that since his visit the president of the university had set aside fifteen hundred dollars to purchase new books for the library and had authorized an increase in the list of periodicals. Dean Long further stated that President Brooks had made available four additional assistant professorships in the departments of the first two years of the School of Medicine and that the president was most keenly interested in the achievement of a class A rating for the school. "If we succeed in the endeavor," Dean Long concluded, "we will all take heart and make the next big drive for a medical school building in Oklahoma City. It is my burning ambition that this school may, in time, be one of the best among the acceptable schools."

Dr. Colwell reported on the inspection of the University of Oklahoma School of Medicine at a meeting of the council on February 29. He informed the council members that unusual improvements had been made during the past two years and that conditions were now fairly acceptable. The council then voted restoration of a class A rating to the school, effective March 1, 1920, on receipt of a definite statement from the president of the university that several deficiencies would be dealt with promptly and that a new college building would definitely be erected at the earliest possible opportunity.

The reinstatement of the School of Medicine to a class A rank was officially announced in a letter of March 11, 1920, from Dr. N. P. Colwell to Dr. Stratton D. Brooks, president of the University of Oklahoma. Dr. Colwell made it crystal clear that the action taken by the council was based on assurances received from the president and the dean that certain other improvements would be brought about in the near future. He urged the president to promote a campaign for these improvements which would include more adequate museum and library facilities, a closer relationship between instruction by the preclinical and clinical departments, fulfillment of the need for special teachers to supervise the work of the senior student clinical clerks in the hospital, better organization of the teaching staffs in the various clinical departments, more detailed announcements concerning medical courses in the catalog, and, finally, recognition of the need for an annual School of Medicine announcement separate from that in the regular university catalog. The most urgent and essential requirement was that a new building be erected to provide better space for laboratories, a library and museum, and administrative offices.

On the same day, March 11, Dr. Colwell wrote a congratulatory letter to Dean LeRoy Long. The letter was richly deserved. There is no question that the achievement of the class A rating was largely due to Governor Williams and Dr. LeRoy Long. As a result of reaching this first goal Dean Long became the leader of the medical profession in Oklahoma and a person who would be known in medical administration throughout the country.

Naturally friends, faculty, and students of the medical school were ecstatically happy about the restored status. The event was celebrated in a full day of activities in Oklahoma City on March 19, 1920. "Our Medical School Into Class A" ran the title of a fervent editorial in the *Journal of the Oklahoma State Medical Association*:

"No happening affecting the Oklahoma doctors, since their organization for mutual betterment, has been received with the very generous acclaim and enthusiasm as was the news, March 18, that our school had been placed in Class A . . . varied sensations of pride and congratulation are felt . . . the long fight to this end, the unreasonable and selfish opposition met from many sources when legislative enactment . . . hung by a thread . . . the strange anomaly of opposition from a few members of the medical profession, inspired by selfishness or pique in the belief that they had met slights in faculty assignments. . . .

"Well, we are through with the first great fight. After this, it will be a matter of increasing pride to build, from the very effective nucleus and organization existing, as great a school as our commercial wealth and resources warrant. The question of lack of money should never again be allowed to harrass the men [to whom] we entrust the great task of building. Above all things, the giving over of control to inferior hands, the baneful influence of political tinkering with a sacred establishment, should be discouraged by every doctor regardless of his political affiliation.

"The maintenance and systematic expansion of every part of this department should have, at all times, the unqualified support of our profession. . . . the maintenance of our school is the concern of all of us; it is not the property of any clique or combination of Oklahoma City physicians, but is the child of the humblest. Its support to the highest point is our concern; its continuous betterment should be the aim of every physician."[1]

The *Journal of the Oklahoma State Medical Association* also reported on the activities on March 19. There were clinics at the University Hospital in the morning, followed by a luncheon for the students and visiting physicians, after which there was a street parade. In the evening more than two hundred physicians and friends attended a banquet at the Skirvin Hotel.

The morning clinics were conducted by Drs. A. B. Chase, C. J. Fishman, J. T. Martin, Lea A. Riely, and A. W. White, medicine; LeRoy Long and A. A. Will, surgery; E. S. Lain, dermatology;

[1] *Journal of the Oklahoma State Medical Association*, Vol. XIII (1920), 151.

E. S. Ferguson, eye, ear, nose, and throat; J. S. Hartford, gynecology; A. D. Young, neurology; and W. J. Wallace, urology.

The University of Oklahoma band headed the afternoon parade, which was made up of highly original floats representing each medical class, the ambulances, and a corps of nurses neatly turned out in uniform. Leonard C. Williams, a medical student, acted as master of ceremonies at the evening banquet. The star of the evening was a junior medical student, Claude Norris, from Le Flore County, Oklahoma. Addresses and comments were made by Drs. LeRoy Long, dean of the faculty; L. A. Turley, assistant dean; A. K. West; Claude A. Thompson, secretary of the Oklahoma State Medical Association; and the Honorable A. N. Leecraft, state treasurer.[2] Governor R. L. Williams, one of the staunch forces in the drive for elevation of the school and for construction of a state hospital, telegraphed his congratulations, saying, "This was due its medical graduates of years gone by, as well as the people of this state."

The 1920 *Journal of the Oklahoma State Medical Association* also carried these reports of two official actions:

Recommendation of Council to House of Delegates

"The membership of the Oklahoma State Medical Association . . . takes this means to congratulate our citizens in every walk of life on:

"First, the establishment of hospital facilities for the medical department of our university which, though now only in an elementary state, has already achieved the award of recognition placing that department in the coveted Class A among the brotherhood of medical schools.

"Second, this association now observes that proper state pride demands that steps be taken to establish a permanent system of orderly increase of the department in exact ratio to the increase of all other departments of the University, in order that the position and class of the department be never humiliated by retrograde

2 *Ibid.*, 154.

decline. . . . in order to adequately render such service, it is necessary for a people to intensely train the medical servant in times of order and peace, and such training must not be on a niggardly, parsimonious scale, but on the scale demanded by the highest efficiency attainable."

Report of Committee on Medical Education, May 20, 1920

"During the last 15 years, there have been remarkable and important advancements in medical education in the United States. Through the activities of the Council on Medical Education of the American Medical Association, the teaching of medicine has been systematized and improved, so that the efficiency of the profession has been greatly increased and people immeasurably benefited. . . .

"Recently the Council on Medical Education of the American Medical Association has advanced the medical department of our State University to A grade. In the judgment of your committee, that action has brought to us not only honor but responsibilities. It should now be our purpose, to not only do what is necessary to retain the coveted A grade, but we should see to it that this department of the University has the necessary support for its proper development. Compared with other states, like Texas, like Iowa, like Michigan, like Virginia, for instance, Oklahoma has contributed but a mere pittance to the development of her School of Medicine. The school has a splendid new hospital, but a great medical building is sorely needed. At present, the first two years work is done at Norman, in inconvenient and inadequate quarters. . . . Your committee strongly recommends that this association urge the next legislature of this state to make an appropriation of $500,000 for the purpose of constructing and equipping the necessary building or buildings for the medical department of the University on the 15 acre tract upon which the State University Hospital is located, and which has been designated by law as the home for the department. Signed by committee members A. L. Blesh, A. K. West, and Arthur W. White."[3]

2 *Ibid.*, 154.

The Council on Medical Education changed its name to the Council on Medical Education and Hospitals in 1920. The first list of hospitals with acceptable internships published by the new council included the University of Oklahoma Hospital and St. Anthony Hospital. The list of schools of medicine[4] in the country included nine two-year schools and seventy-six four-year schools, of which seventy were in class A, seven in class B, and eight in class C.[5]

In 1920, Dr. Wann Langston was appointed medical superintendent of the University Hospital; Paul Fesler remained the fiscal superintendent and chief clerk, with Dean Long the chief administrator. Esther Grace Bayles became dietitian for the hospital, and a position of pharmacist was added to the budget. Apparently there were no written bylaws pertaining to the University Hospital at the time.

At the June 6 faculty meeting that year, Dean Long announced that Dr. Basil Hayes and Dr. Walker Morledge, interns at the Cleveland City Hospital, had accepted positions as residents at the University Hospital. There were also places for five interns on the staff. Beginning in 1920 the interns were under the supervision of residents on duty in the hospital. The general outpatient clinic remained at the Emergency Hospital building at Third and Stiles streets, and the number of patients at this clinic was said to have averaged 150 a day.

The official schedule of charges at the University Hospital in 1920 was: private room, $5 to $7 a day and ward bed, $15 a week, with special fees for operating room, laboratory, and so on. In a letter dated October, 1920, Dean Long wrote that it was the practice of most hospitals to make a discount to physicians and clergymen when they were patients at the hospital and that the University Hospital had had for some time an unwritten regulation allowing a discount of 20 per cent to physicians, surgeons, and minor children of their families. It was his opinion that the discount should not be so large that it would reduce the bill below

4 Five homeopathic, one eclectic, and three nondescript schools were on the list.
5 *Journal of the American Medical Association*, Vol. LXXV (1920), 381, 396.

the amount of money actually expended by the hospital in the care of the patient, and he felt that most physicians would hesitate to ask a hospital to render them a service without any payment at all.

There were seventy-three faculty members in the School of Medicine during the academic year 1920–21. The following new members were appointed in 1920: Joseph Mario Thuringer, M.D., professor of histology and embryology; John Zell Gaston, B.S., assistant professor of anatomy; Hiram Dunlap Moor, M.S., assistant professor of bacteriology; Alma Jessie Neill, Ph.D., assistant professor of physiology; Merlin Jones Stone, B.S., assistant professor of anatomy; Ray Morton Balyeat, M.D., instructor in medicine; Charles Nelson Berry, M.D., instructor in surgery; John Lewis Day, M.D., instructor in physical diagnosis and minor surgery; James Jackson Gable, M.D., instructor in mental diseases and medical jurisprudence; John Evans Heatley, M.D., instructor in dermatology, electrotherapy, and radiography; Thomas Claude Lowry, M.D., instructor in medicine; Walter Howard Miles, M.D., instructor in medicine; Raymond Lester Murdoch, M.D., instructor in surgery; and Elba Kenneth Mabry, D.D.S., dentist outpatient department.

At a meeting of the faculty on June 6, President Stratton Brooks presided and reported that he had recommended separate appropriations for the University Medical School and for the University Hospital. A motion was passed that the dean appoint a committee to plan development of postgraduate courses for the school and hospital.

Dean LeRoy Long made his annual report, including an announcement of the advancement of the school to grade A by the Council on Medical Education. He advised the faculty of the recommendations for further improvements made by Dr. Colwell and emphasized the need for a new building to provide more generous space for laboratories, the library, and administrative offices.

Dean Long then told of the attempt to gain appropriations to construct a medical school building. "At this time, we are endeavoring to lay the foundation for a campaign in connection with

155

securing an appropriation of $500,000 for the purpose of constructing a building for the medical school. I am glad to be able to report that the Oklahoma State Medical Association, at its recent meeting in Oklahoma City, went on record in connection with this important matter, the House of Delegates adopting, without a dissenting vote, the report of its Committee on Education.

"In my judgment, the adoption of the above report by the unanimous vote of the House of Delegates of the state association is of the greatest importance at this time, as it places organized medicine of this state on record in favor of such an appropriation by the Legislature."

There were two other faculty meetings in 1920. At the October 11 meeting, with Dr. Long presiding, a resolution was passed in memory of Dr. John W. Duke, professor of mental diseases, 1915–20.

A new Department of Histology and Embryology was formed in 1920, with Dr. Joseph Mario Thuringer as its head. This was the last year during which anesthesia was taught under the Department of Surgery. It was transferred to the Department of Medicine in 1921. It appears that the course known as pharmaceutical methods was terminated during the year.

A second national medical fraternity, Alpha Kappa Kappa, was established at the University of Oklahoma School of Medicine in 1920. In that year fifteen graduates of the School of Medicine received the M.D. degree. Among them were Clarence Edgar Bates, Carl Langley Brundage, and Warren Troutman Mayfield. Twelve graduates of the Training School for Nurses received G.N. certificates. During the 1920–21 academic year there were 103 students in the School of Medicine and 38 in the Training School for Nurses. The fees in the School of Medicine for the four years were $70, $40, $40, and $45, respectively.

The 1920–21 university catalog reported a total of $891,392 for support of the university during that year, with $73,060 for the University Hospital and an additional $14,281 for buildings.

In 1921 the American Legion demanded of the eighth legislature that something be done to provide disabled servicemen with immediate hospital facilities. The legislature responded by providing $75,000 to build an adjoining administrative wing at the University Hospital. This made it possible to equip a ward for servicemen on the hospital's third floor.[6] Additional appropriations were made as follows: for a nurses' home, $60,000; equipment, $37,500; and remodeling, $10,000. This brought the total investment in the University Hospital to approximately $450,000 and provided an additional 28,000 square feet of much-needed floor space.

During the eighth legislative session two separate bills were passed which could have caused considerable embarrassment to the School of Medicine due to a lack of effective team work and communication between the legislative committee of the Oklahoma State Medical Association and the authorities of the school. These bills provided for two new separate boards, a State Board of Osteopathy (the Oklahoma Osteopathic Act) and a board named Chiropractic Examiners. The osteopathic act, as proposed, was an apparent attempt to gain entrance to the faculty of the School of Medicine of the university and to the staffs of state or city hospitals within the jurisdiction of the state. The Oklahoma State Medical Association was properly disturbed by this aggression as attested by various letters in the files of the office of the dean. However, since the State Board of Medical Examiners was ineffective in modifying the osteopathic act, members of the faculty of the School of Medicine assumed the responsibility of rectifying the situation and took active steps to forestall what might have become a very embarrassing confrontation for their school. The bill was recalled from the governor's desk, where it had gone after passage by both houses, and the particular section which would have been

6 The May 2, 1969 issue of the *Daily Oklahoman* carried an article entitled "Legion Celebrates 50 years." Hugh P. Haugherty, department historian, was quoted as saying, "The people of Oklahoma in all these years have been very good to the veterans." He recalled that the first benefit for veterans came shortly after the legion's founding, when officials of the University Hospital were attempting to build a new wing. "They told us that if we would help them in getting the addition they would set aside 100 beds for veterans. The addition was won, and the hospital kept its word."

157

exceedingly troublesome for the School of Medicine was deleted from the bill.

The building program in 1921 included construction of the nurses' home adjacent to the west wing of the hospital and the remodeling of an area for dispensary quarters in the new University Hospital, so that certain functions of the outpatient department could be moved there. The bed capacity of the new hospital was increased from 176 to approximately 276 beds, and a Social Service Department was established, with Virginia Tolbert as the first social service worker. Miss Tolbert formed an advisory council of five interested women in Oklahoma City to assist in developing the department. She later became Mrs. William Alonzo Fowler. Dr. H. B. Rigby was appointed resident in surgery, and Dr. Clark H. Hall was appointed resident in medicine that year.

There were two faculty meetings in 1921. President Brooks presided at the June 4 meeting when Dean Long reported improvement in the student body due to the advanced requirements for entrance and the restoration of the school to class A, which had resulted in a remarkable increase in applications. Dean Long went on record as favoring foreign language requirements for medical students. He also praised Paul Fesler for his fine work in helping to secure appropriations for the School of Medicine.

During April, 1921, Dean Long advised Medical Superintendent Wann Langston that he was constantly receiving complaints from referring physicians that no information was being sent to them in regard to the condition of their referred patients. This unsatisfactory state of affairs was to reappear on various occasions over a period of three decades due to insufficient clerical staff, a result of the limited appropriations by the legislature.

At the second faculty meeting, on July 13, Dean Long reported that the University Hospital now had a well-equipped laboratory, an electrocardiograph, and a metabolism unit and that there had been improvements in the x-ray equipment. He stated further that he had just returned from the annual meeting of the Congress on Medical Education, where it was the majority opinion that the first two years of medical training should not be separated geographically from the last two years. He recommended that a fifth or hospital year be required for licensing. Dean Long mentioned, incidentally, that the National Board of Medical Examiners had been originally organized in 1915. In a closing comment he said, "It goes without saying that the Council on Medical Education does not expect us to stand still."

There were seventy-one faculty members of the School of Medicine in the 1921–22 academic year. The only faculty member added during 1921 was Richard Clyde Lowry, M.D., instructor in obstetrics.

In October, Helen Kendall was employed as secretary to the dean and faculty and as clerk of the clinic. Her title became Clerk of the Medical School in 1922. She was given general charge of the library in Oklahoma City until 1928, when the new School of Medicine building was constructed there.

The 1921–22 bulletin of the School of Medicine stated that the maternity work was conducted in the University Hospital and the Holmes Home of Redeeming Love. At that time St. Anthony Hospital, a teaching affiliate, still had a capacity of 130 beds.

The appropriations available for the support of the University Hospital during 1921–22 were, according to the 1921–22 university catalog, $125,000 for salaries, $52,520 for maintenance, $102,500 for soldiers' relief, and $1,500 for nurses' quarters—a total of $281,520, with the following additional amounts for permanent improvements: $25,000 for hospital equipment, $20,000 for radium, and $1,000 for soldiers' relief. The support for the university that year was $949,252. The fees for medical students, according to the 1921 *Journal of the American Medical Association*, were $60, $60, $25, and $25 for the four classes.[7]

Seventeen graduates received the M.D. degree in 1921. Included were Charles Leonard Brown,[8] Ben Hunter Cooley, James Burnette Eskridge, Jr., Ellis Moore, and Theodore Grant Wails. Twelve nursing graduates received the certificate of G.N. During

[7] *Journal of the American Medical Association*, Vol. LXXVII (1921), 529.

[8] Dr. Charles L. Brown, a distinguished graduate of the School of Medicine, was later dean of the Hahnemann Medical College in Philadelphia, Pennsylvania, and then of the Seton Hall College of Medicine, in Jersey City, New Jersey.

the academic year 1921–22 there were 117 students in the School of Medicine and 46 students in the Training School for Nurses. A third professional medical fraternity, Chi Zeta Chi, and the Alumni Association of the University of Oklahoma School of Nursing were organized at the university in 1921.

On March 3, 1922, an article on the University Hospital appeared in *Harlow's Weekly* which contained many interesting observations and comments concerning the development of the School of Medicine—its finances, building program, and administration. "In point of building facilities and equipment," the article stated, "the University Hospital is easily the best hospital in Oklahoma, and is one of the best state university hospitals in the nation. The only thing the Department of Medicine of the University of Oklahoma needs to complete its equipment is a new medical school building, on the hospital grounds at Oklahoma City, to provide classrooms and laboratory facilities for the students who are now forced to take the first two years of the medical course in inadequate quarters at the University of Oklahoma in Norman."[9]

It was estimated in the article that by March the University Hospital addition would be ready for occupancy and the second floor of the main hospital building remodeled to provide 100 more beds for patients (in addition to the present 185 beds) which would take care of the soldiers until such time as the new federal hospital could be opened in Muskogee. It should be stated here that the Soldiers Relief Commission of the state, the American Legion, the Red Cross, and other welfare organizations had been very co-operative in regard to the remodeling of the University Hospital.

In the article in *Harlow's Weekly* it was further stated that "the Department of Medicine of the University would not mean so much to the state were it not for the influence of Dr. Long. In Oklahoma the position of Dean of the State Medical School means much more than in other states. Here, he not only conducts his school but he also largely shapes the course of his profession, establishes the medical ethics of his state and acts as the leader of his associates

[9] *Harlow's Weekly*, Vol. XXI (March 3, 1922), 11.

and students in the medical profession. . . . In Oklahoma, according to a report of the American College of Surgeons, there are only two fully equipped hospitals, the University Hospital and St. Anthony Hospital, both in Oklahoma City.[10] All these factors make it necessary that the Dean of Oklahoma Medical School be a true representative of his profession, gifted with unusual qualities and of proven ability. Dr. Long seems to have these requirements. . . . The University Hospital cannot be understood without understanding Dr. Long—he is the heart of it. For seven years, he has given the best of his life to the school and the dreams and hopes he has had for the institution have been realized in greater degree each year as the school has grown. . . . The official family of the hospital is composed of Dean LeRoy Long, Superintendent Paul Fesler, Medical Superintendent Dr. Wann Langston, 55 Oklahoma City physicians, and those connected with the first two years of the School of Medicine at Norman. There are in the hospital ten house staff members who are graduates from medical schools all over the United States, 20 graduate nurses, and [46] student nurses. . . . The School of Medicine is subject to Dr. Brooks, President of the University of Oklahoma, but it is directly under the supervision of Dr. LeRoy Long. Dr. Brooks has little to do with the administrative work of the Medical School, except in an advisory way, as this work is left to Dr. Long. Paul Fesler, the Superintendent, has charge of the fiscal affairs of the hospital. The state appropriates only $175,000 a year for maintenance and equipment of the University Hospital, which is about $100,000 a year less than is necessary to do the work required. Therefore, it is necessary for the hospital to produce enough revenue through fees to meet this deficit. The physicians who constitute the staff of the hospital do not collect any fees from the charity patients."[11]

The article indicates that interns received $25 a month and student nurses $8 to $15 a week, while graduate nurses were paid

[10] On March 20, 1922, the regents authorized the University Hospital to join the American Hospital Association.

[11] *Harlow's Weekly*, Vol. XXI (March 3, 1922), 11.

salaries commensurate with their particular services.[12] There were three classes of patients at the University Hospital, namely, clinical, semiprivate, and private. A charge of $15 a week for hospitalization was in effect in 1922, and there were twenty rooms for private patients in the hospital.

In operation at the time was a gratuity made possible by the medical staff through contribution of their fees from private patients. This fund was known as the Doctors Fund. It was managed by the medical staff for the purpose of buying special equipment for the hospital.

In a report of the University Hospital for the year ending June 30, 1922, Dr. Long's title was given as dean of the School of Medicine and chief of staff of University Hospital. In the same report it was stated that the administrative wing was completed May 1, and that all administrative departments of the hospital were then moved from the main building. The basements were used for a central storeroom, kitchens, and dining rooms. The main floor of the new wing housed the administrative offices, a consultation room, and a reception room. The second floor contained the library for the house staff, classrooms, and rooms for interns; the third floor was entirely taken up by laboratories, which had been greatly improved by additional new equipment. In the main hospital the first floor was being remodeled to be used for children, adult male surgery, the social service department, and the receiving room.

Modern quarters for the school for nurses were also constructed during the year, making provision for classrooms, a library, demonstration room, and reception room, as well as dormitory rooms for the nursing students. As stated previously, this new building was erected adjacent to the west wing of the University Hospital.

In a report by the superintendent of the University Hospital on July 1, 1922, the need for a new school of medicine building at the Oklahoma City campus was stressed. Paul Fesler indicated also

---

[12] Other salaries were: superintendent of the hospital, $3,600; medical director, $3,600; superintendent of nurses, $2,400; and residents, $1,200. Helen Kendall received $1,620 a year as medical school clerk.

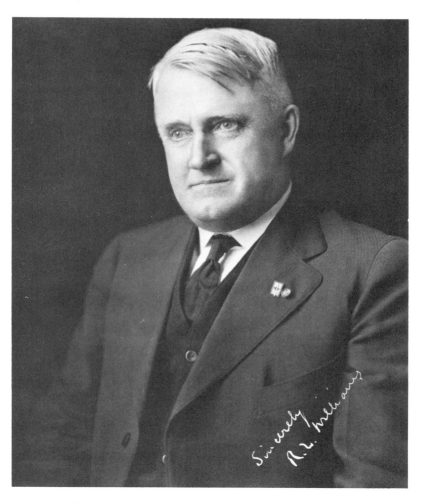

Governor Robert Lee Williams, the third governor of Oklahoma, proved to be an able friend of the University of Oklahoma School of Medicine. His continued support of the medical school greatly contributed to its growth and improvement.

Courtesy Oklahoma Historical Society

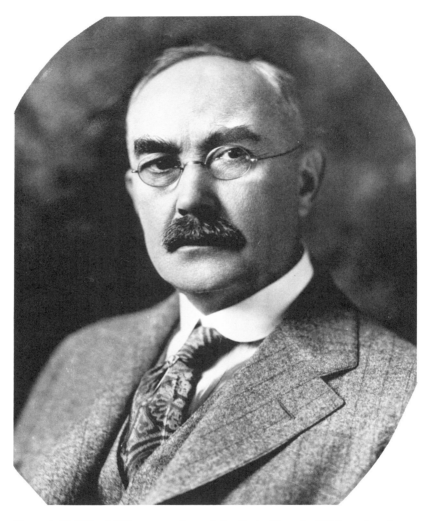

Francis B. Fite, M.D., a member of the State Board of Education from 1913 to 1919, was a strong supporter of the School of Medicine.

Courtesy Mrs. Hubert Ambrister

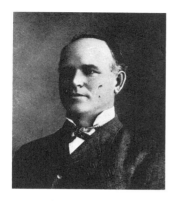

Albert Heald Van Vleet, Ph.D., head of the Department of Biology, 1898–1909.

Courtesy Sooner Yearbook

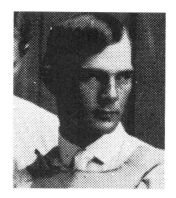

Walter L. Capshaw, M.D., head of the Department of Anatomy, 1908–15.

Courtesy Sooner Yearbook

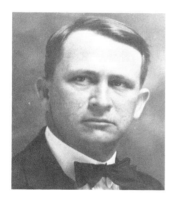

Reuben M. Hargrove, M.D., head of the Department of Anatomy, 1916–19.

Courtesy Oklahoma State Board of Medical Examiners

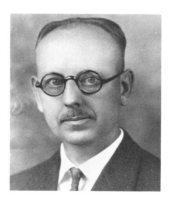

Joseph C. Stephenson, Ph.D., M.D., head of the Department of Anatomy, 1919–31.

Courtesy Oklahoma State Board of Medical Examiners

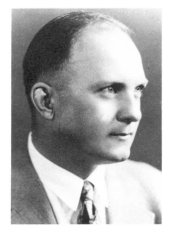

Carmen R. Salsbury, M.D., head of the Department of Anatomy, 1931–33.

Courtesy Salsbury family

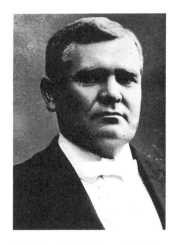

Edwin C. DeBarr, Ph.D., head of the Department of Chemistry, 1906–23.

Courtesy Sooner Yearbook

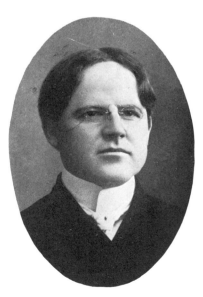

Edward Marsh Williams, B.S., head of the Department of Pathology and Bacteriology, 1906–1908.

Courtesy Mistletoe

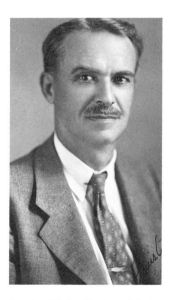

Louis Alvin Turley, M.A., head of the Department of Pathology and Bacteriology, 1909–44.

Courtesy Sooner Medic

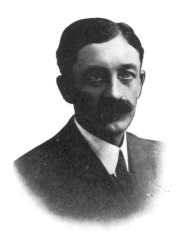

John Dice Maclaren, M.D., head of the Department of Physiology, 1908–11.

Courtesy Sooner Yearbook

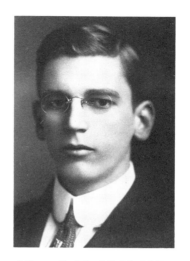

Albert C. Hirshfield, M.D., head of the Department of Physiology, 1911–12.

Courtesy Oklahoma State Board of Medical Examiners

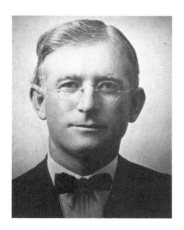

Leonard B. Nice, Ph.D., head of the Department of Physiology, 1913–27.

Courtesy Nice family

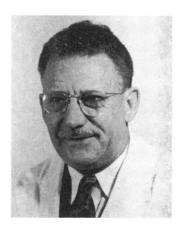

Edward C. Mason, Ph.D., M.D., head of the Department of Physiology, 1928–50.

Courtesy Sooner Medic

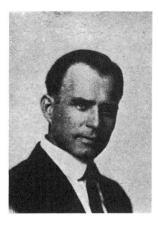

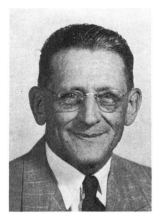

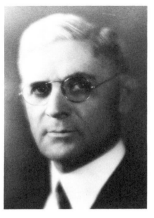

Gayfree Ellison, M.D., head of the Department of Bacteriology and Hygiene, 1912–28, and head of the Department of Preventive Medicine, 1912–32.

Courtesy Sooner Yearbook

Hiram D. Moor, M.S., head of the Department of Bacteriology, 1929–51.

Courtesy Sooner Medic

William J. Wallace, M.D., head of the Department of Urology, 1919–34.

Courtesy Mrs. William J. Hefner

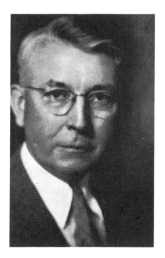

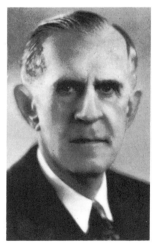

John W. Riley, M.D., head of the Department of Surgery, 1913–15, and head of the Department of Urology, 1913–19.

Courtesy Oklahoma City Academy of Medicine

Robert M. Howard, M.D., head of the Department of Surgery, 1931–43.

Courtesy Oklahoma City Academy of Medicine

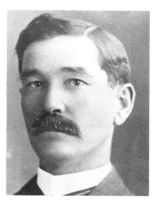

Archa Kelly West, M.D., dean of the Epworth College of Medicine and head of the Department of Medicine, University of Oklahoma School of Medicine, 1912–26.

Courtesy University of Oklahoma Medical Center

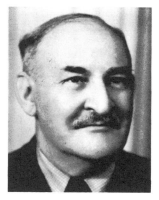

George A. LaMotte, M.D., head of the Department of Medicine, 1926–44.

Courtesy Oklahoma City Academy of Medicine

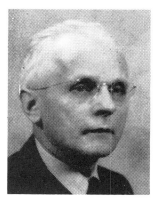

Joseph Mario Thuringer, M.D., head of Department of Histology and Embryology, 1920–50.

Courtesy Sooner Medic

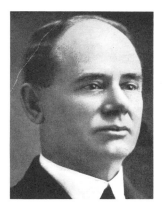

John S. Hartford, M.D., director of the outpatient staff, 1912–14, and head of the Department of Gynecology, 1916–24.

Courtesy Oklahoma City Academy of Medicine

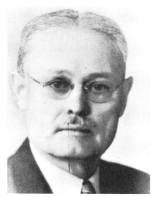

John F. Kuhn, M.D., head of the Department of Gynecology, 1924–39.

Courtesy Oklahoma City Academy of Medicine

169

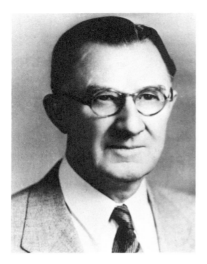

Everett S. Lain, M.D., head of the Department of Radiology, 1911–36, and head of the Department of Dermatology, 1916–42.

Courtesy University of Oklahoma Medical Center

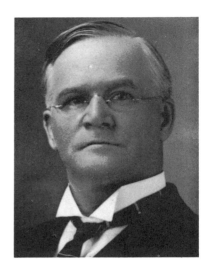

John A. Hatchett, M.D., head of the Department of Obstetrics, 1912–33.

Courtesy Oklahoma City Academy of Medicine

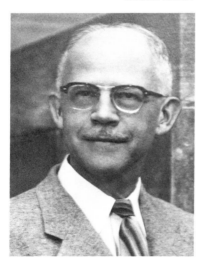

Mark R. Everett, Ph.D., head of the Department of Biochemistry, 1924–64.

Courtesy University of Oklahoma Medical Center

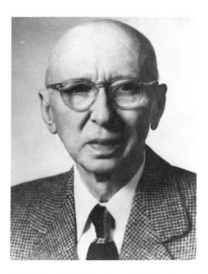

William M. Taylor, M.D., head of the Department of Pediatrics, 1930–38.

Courtesy Mrs. Paul L. Moore

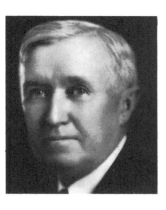
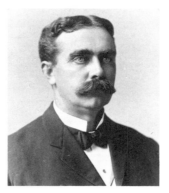
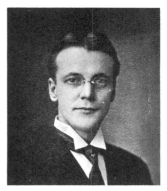

Edmund S. Ferguson, M.D., head of the Department of Ophthalmology, 1912–38.

Courtesy Oklahoma City Academy of Medicine

Lauren H. Buxton, M.D., head of the Department of Otorhinolaryngology, 1916–21.

Courtesy University of Oklahoma Medical Center

Harry Coulter Todd, M.D., head of the Department of Otorhinolaryngology, 1924–30.

Courtesy Sooner Yearbook

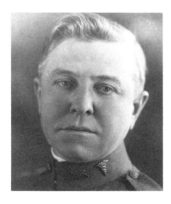
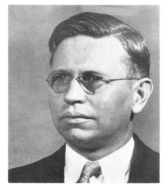

Floyd Bolend, M.D., emeritus head of the Department of Anesthesiology, 1930–37.

Courtesy Mrs. Horace Thompson

John A. Moffett, M.D., head of the Department of Anesthesiology, 1930–38.

Courtesy Oklahoma State Board of Medical Examiners

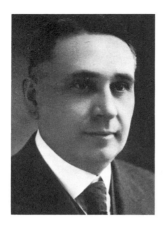 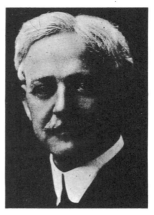 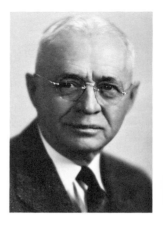

Antonio D. Young, M.D., head of the Department of Psychiatry and Neurology, 1912–15.

Courtesy Oklahoma City Academy of Medicine

John W. Duke, M.D., head of the Department of Psychiatry and Neurology, 1916–19.

Courtesy Journal of the Oklahoma State Medical Association

David W. Griffin, M.D., head of the Department of Psychiatry and Neurology, 1920–40.

Courtesy Russell Smith

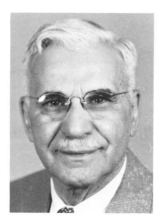 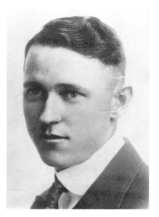

Casriel J. Fishman, M.D., head of the Department of Neurology, 1930–46.

Courtesy University of Oklahoma Medical Center

James J. Gable, M.D., acting head of the Department of Neurology, 1930.

Courtesy Oklahoma State Board of Medical Examiners

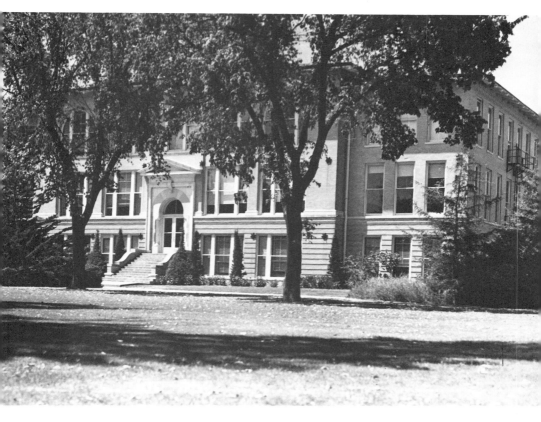

Science Hall, on the university campus in Norman, where medical
school classes were taught.

Courtesy Sooner Medic

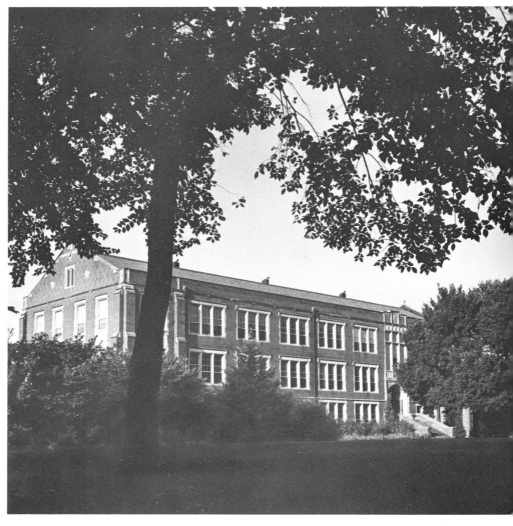

The second School of Medicine building on the University of Oklahoma campus in Norman, 1924.

Courtesy Sooner Medic

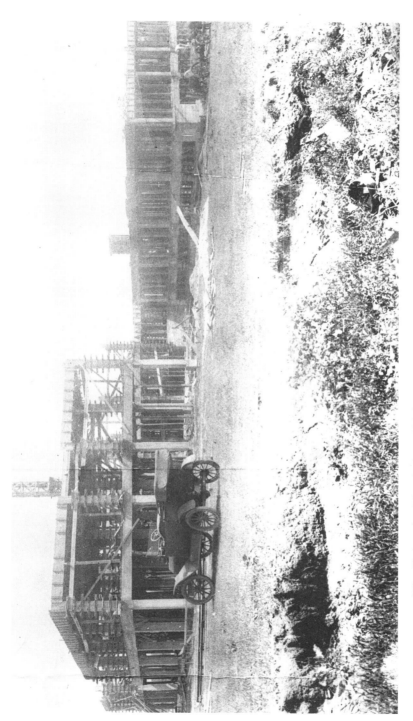

The University Hospital in Oklahoma City under construction, 1918.

Courtesy University of Oklahoma Medical Center

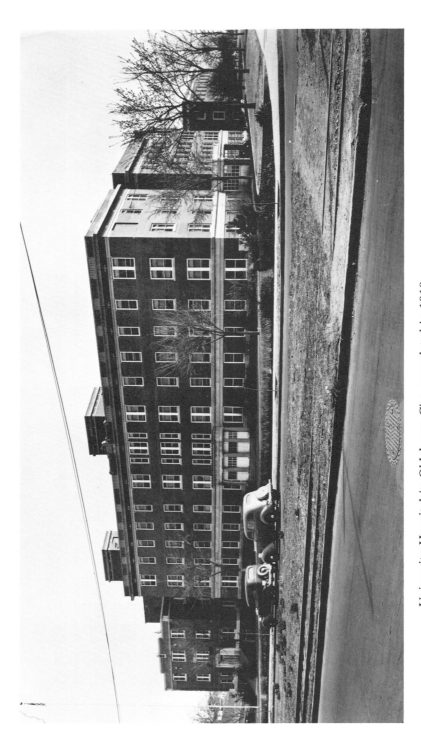

University Hospital in Oklahoma City, completed in 1919.

Courtesy University of Oklahoma Medical Center

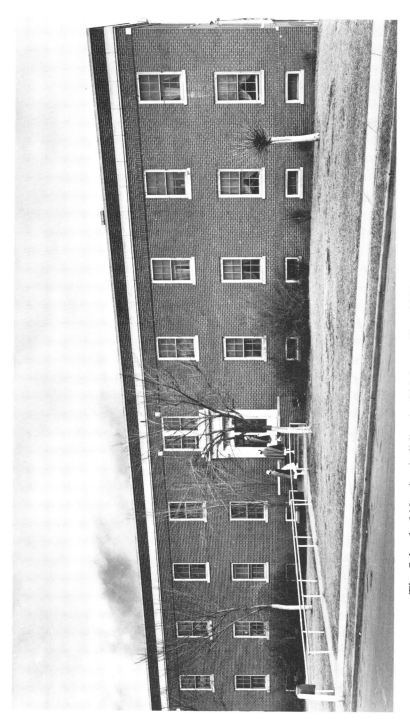

The School of Nursing building in Oklahoma City, 1921.

Courtesy University of Oklahoma Medical Center

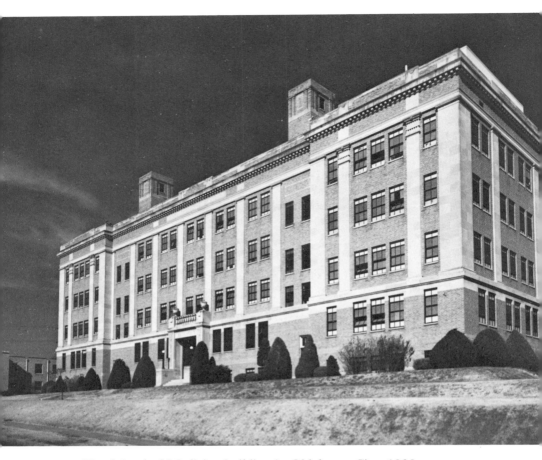

The School of Medicine building in Oklahoma City, 1928.

Courtesy University of Oklahoma Medical Center

that a 150-bed hospital building for children was essential, as well as a power plant and a considerably enlarged nurses home.

Fesler also stated that the school for nurses had been greatly improved and that the number of applicants for admission to it had increased since completion of the Nurses Home with its added teaching facilities. Fesler said that Candice Monfort, superintendent of nurses, had been wonderfully successful in her efforts to improve the status of the School of Nursing, which had achieved its own class A rating.

Mr. Fesler expressed gratitude to Dr. Wann Langston for his "untiring efforts to maintain proper patient care and for a greatly improved intern service under his management." The hospital laboratories, also under the administration of Dr. Langston, had been improved considerably since occupation of the new quarters and installation of new equipment. The 1922 annual report of the work of these laboratories showed the following numbers of determinations: serological laboratory, 3,361; x-ray laboratory, 1,891; blood chemistry, 2,144; special chemistry, 1,118; tissue pathology, 465; bacteriology laboratory, 3,641; and in the clinical laboratory, 7,358 urine examinations, 5,612 blood examinations, and 128 cerebrospinal fluid and ascitic fluid examinations. There were 150 tests in the basal metabolism laboratory and 159 in the electro-cardiograph laboratory.

In 1922 there was a hospital board with Dr. E. S. Ferguson as chairman, the other members being Dr. Lea Riely, Dr. A. W. White, Dr. W. J. Wallace, Dr. J. S. Hartford, and Dean Long, ex-officio. The house staff of ten included the two residents and eight interns. Among the latter were Dr. Elmer R. Musick, Dr. Ephraim Goldfain, and Dr. Ben H. Cooley.

In the first annual report (November, 1922) of the new Social Service Department, instituted at the University Hospital on November 11, 1921, Paul Fesler expressed the belief that the department should be affiliated with the Social Service Department on the Norman campus of the university, so that students there could receive practical work in hospital social service. Miss Tolbert

179

expressed appreciation for the opening of a special school for crippled children in Oklahoma City, which enabled the hospital to bring certain additional crippled children to the hospital from all parts of the state. Eight children had already begun attending this school. Alberta Webb and Lois Jones were appointed salaried teachers for the school.

Other statistics for the University Hospital in 1921 and 1922 were as follows: patients admitted during the year ending June 30, 1921, 2,983, and during the year ending June 30, 1922, 3,725; the corresponding numbers of days of patient treatment during these two years were 44,923 in 1921 and 48,709 in 1922. The average number of days of hospitalization for each patient was fifteen in 1921 and thirteen in 1922. Two thousand and forty patients were admitted to the dispensary during the year ending June, 1921, and 3,499 during the year ending June 30, 1922. The number of treatment days in the dispensary for 1921 was 14,696, and for 1922, 27,711.

Concerning revenue, the university catalog for 1922–23 stated that the University Hospital had received $125,000 for salaries, $52,500 for maintenance, $22,500 for salaries for soldiers' relief, $80,000 for maintenance of the same enterprise, and a general revenue of $1,000 for maintenance, making a total appropriation of $281,000. The support for the university was $939,252.

President Brooks presided at a faculty meeting on June 2, 1922, at which he stated that the assets of the School of Medicine amounted to $578,000, all acquired since 1917. "More than half a million in five years is not so bad," said he.

There were seventy-seven members of the faculty in the School of Medicine during the academic year, 1922–23. Those who were newly appointed in 1922 were: Esther Grace Bayles, dietitian and instructor in dietetics; Ben Hunter Cooley, M.D., instructor in minor surgery; Clark Homer Hall, M.D., instructor in pediatrics; Basil Augustus Hayes, M.D., instructor in surgery; Carroll Monroe Pounders, M.D., instructor in pediatrics; Theodore Grant Wails, M.D., instructor in ophthalmology; Mallalieu McCullagh Wickham, M.A., instructor in histology, embryology, and zoology; Wilbert James Scruton, D.D.S., consultant in dental surgery; and B. Louise Bond, R.N., assistant superintendent of nurses. Dr. Lauren Haynes Buxton became professor emeritus of otology, rhinology, and laryngology in 1922, and Dr. E. S. Ferguson was made head of a temporary joint Department of Ophthalmology, Otology, Rhinology, and Laryngology, an arrangement which continued until 1924.

Fifteen graduates of the school received the M.D. degree in 1922. In this graduating class were Norphleete Price Eley, Hugh Clifford Jones, and Richard Gray Soutar. There were 140 medical students enrolled in the School of Medicine during the academic year 1922–23. This was the year in which the Phi Chi professional medical fraternity was founded at the School of Medicine.

The G.N. certificate was awarded to ten graduating students of the Training School for Nurses in 1922, and there were forty-seven students in the school during the academic year. The superintendent of nurses, Candice Monfort, felt that the completion of the new nurses' home had been the greatest event in the school during the year. She said the number of applications for training had increased and the quality of the applicants showed marked improvement.

Selected abstracts from the annual report of the dean of the School of Medicine to the president of the University of Oklahoma for the year ending June 30, 1922, provide an excellent summary for this period.

"The school was advanced to an A grade institution a short time after the commencement of active work in the hospital. Without the hospital it could not exist as a school of the first class. On the other hand, without the School of Medicine, it would not be possible to render free service to the poor people of the state on a comprehensive scale, for it is through well-organized teaching institutions only that such service can be rendered.

"Before the completion of the hospital, our greatest problem was to secure patients for clinical teaching. Now the situation is reversed, our present problem being to keep up the organization of the School of Medicine in such a way that the increasing number

181

of poor people coming to us from every part of the state may be cared for properly.

"At present, the School of Medicine is geographically divided, half of the time being spent at Norman and half at Oklahoma City. In order to have the greatest efficiency possible—an efficiency which the increasing work of the hospital demands—it is necessary to have the school united.

"The School of Medicine is growing very rapidly. It is attracting students from various parts of the nation and some from foreign countries, but on account of the lack of room, many of those applying cannot be admitted.

"We have no permanent home at Norman. There the school is housed in a cheap wooden building and in some rooms in old Science Hall that are sorely needed by other departments of the University. Practically, we have nothing at Norman except the personnel and moveable apparatus. At Oklahoma City, we have 15 acres of land designated by law as the home for the Medical Department of the University.

"At this time, notwithstanding a bed capacity of 276, the hospital is taxed in the effort to care for the indigent citizens of the state coming to it. In order to carry on the work so that none will be denied admittance, the facilities should be increased. In addition to the medical building, we ought to have a children's building, a combined power house and laundry, and a new nurses home—the present inadequate house being converted into quarters for infectious and contagious diseases. The original hospital building and the administration building should be completed. Since, however, the work of the hospital is so distinctly predicated upon the School of Medicine, any increase of hospital space would be useless without the medical building through which the school would remain an A grade institution, and its activities be unified in such a way that a greater service could be rendered through the hospital.

"It is the desire of those of us connected with the School of Medicine to not only perform our duties in such a way as to retain the coveted A rating, but to make it one of the great medical institutions of the country. With these things in mind, I have endeavored to point out some of our needs, the most urgent being, in my judgment, the construction and equipment of the medical building on the land set apart in connection with the University Hospital at Oklahoma City as a home for the school. Obediently yours, LeRoy Long, Dean of the School of Medicine."

X. The First School of Medicine Building and Postgraduate Instruction: 1923–26

JOHN C. WALTON, mayor of Oklahoma City, ran for governor of Oklahoma on a radical platform in 1922, and was elected by a huge majority. Born in Indiana in 1881, Walton had moved to Nebraska and subsequently to Oklahoma Territory as an engineer. His term as fifth governor of the state was destined to be short and full of trouble, including a major collision with the second Ku Klux Klan, then at the peak of its political power.

Governor Walton regarded the governor's office as a sort of patronage center. Soon after being sworn in he began to tamper with the University of Oklahoma and the Oklahoma Agricultural and Mechanical College in an effort to secure favors through their governing boards and to put pressure on their presidents and faculty members. These unconscionable actions resulted in the resignation of President Brooks on July 1, 1923, after the governor had removed most of the university regents and replaced them with new appointees. Similar events at the Oklahoma Agricultural and Mechanical College resulted in the resignation of President J. B. Eskridge on August 4, 1923.

Popular opposition to Governor Walton built rapidly. It grew so intense that his term, which had begun January 9, 1923, ended with his impeachment on November 19 of the same year. Walton had already been suspended on October 23, making Lieutenant Governor Martin Edwin Trapp the acting governor of the state until November 19, when he became the chief executive. Trapp proved to be a conservative and able governor, sincerely interested in the welfare of the university.

Dean LeRoy Long wrote a letter, dated June 18, 1923, to Dr. N. P. Colwell, secretary of the Council on Medical Education and Hospitals, in which he states that it was well understood that President Stratton D. Brooks had resigned because of political interference which had made it impossible for him to remain and that the alumni of the university were very bitter about the whole affair. Dr. Brooks promptly left Oklahoma to assume the duties of president of the University of Missouri, in his native state. Emissaries from the University of Missouri had been entreating him to accept this position for some time. Upon the resignation of President Brooks, Dr. James S. Buchanan became acting president of the University of Oklahoma, and in July, 1924, Dr. Buchanan was elected president of the university.

While the medical faculty shared the concern over the actions of Governor Walton, apparently the School of Medicine did not suffer greatly during his short tenure of office. On the contrary, the ninth legislature enacted a very important piece of legislation in the passage of Senate Bill No. 311, entitled Medical Treatment of Children.[1] This bill provided for medical and surgical treatment of children with remediable maladies, when their parents were unable to provide such treatment. Children in this category were to be committed to the University Hospital by the juvenile courts, with the parents' consent, and no compensation was chargeable under the law by physician, surgeon, or nurse. The hospital fee, not to exceed fifteen dollars a week, was the responsibility of the county in which the patient lived. The medical faculty of the University Hospital was required to prepare the necessary blanks for the medical examination, under order of the court.

Two members of the House of Representatives, Allen M. Street, an Oklahoma City Rotarian, and James C. Nance, of Stephens County, secured the enactment of this first state law for the medical care of indigent crippled children. Paul Fesler, also a Rotarian and

[1] *Session Laws*, 1923, Chapter 105, 172.

the superintendent of the University Hospital, sponsored the bill, which was passed and signed by Governor Walton. The Rotary Club was also instrumental in forming the Oklahoma Society for Crippled Children.[2]

The ninth legislature also passed House Bill No. 15, appropriating $100,000 for a building on the campus in Norman to house the preclinical instruction of the School of Medicine. In a subsequent special session the legislature confirmed this appropriation.[3] The 1923–24 appropriation for the operation of the University Hospital was $275,000, and the support for the rest of the university was $1,042,825.

The legislature, in appropriating the above fund for a medical building at Norman, very obviously had not heeded the advice and judgment of the medical school administration that the new building should be located on the Oklahoma City campus.

Dean Long had expressed himself on this matter on several occasions and reiterated his position once more when he wrote, "We should—we must—have the broader and higher view and build here a great institution that will serve not only Oklahoma but the world, for in doing this, Oklahoma will be better served." Continuing, Dean Long said, "At present, the School of Medicine is geographically divided, the first two years being at Norman, and the last two years at Oklahoma City. This is a great misfortune. . . . medical educators are unanimous in the belief that all four years should be at the same place for the good of the students. . . . the student grows into the profession rather than being suddenly thrown into it after two years of classroom work in which he is unable to see the relation that should exist between it and the practical work of the profession for which he is preparing him-

2 For histories of early crippled children laws in Oklahoma, see the *First Annual Report of the Oklahoma Commission for Crippled Children* (Oklahoma City, Oklahoma Commission for Crippled Children, 1936), 4–7, and Earl D. McBride, M.D., "The Oklahoma Society for Crippled Children," *Chronicles of Oklahoma*, Vol. XXVII, No. 2 (1949), 170–78. The Crippled Children's Committee of the Oklahoma City Rotary Club was formed in 1920, with Walter C. Dean as chairman. On this committee were five lay citizens and Drs. C. N. Gould, Everett S. Lain, Earl D. McBride, Horace Reed, and T. Wallace Sorrels.

3 *Special Session Laws*, 1923–24, Chapter 102, 118.

self. . . . The better medical schools of the country are now holding clinics for the benefit of freshmen and sophomore students. . . . With the school geographically divided, it is not possible for the faculties of the two ends to have free coordination. . . . The object of this article is to the end that the medical profession of this state may be truthfully advised, and being advised, assist us in every proper way to build here in Oklahoma a great medical school which shall be known not only in our own state, but throughout the nation, not only at home, but abroad."[4]

Commenting on the medical school's hospitals, in the same article, Dean Long reported that the outpatient clinic at Third and Stiles Streets was caring for an average of 100 to 150 patients daily and that on several occasions the new University Hospital had accommodated more than 300 patients at one time. Practically all patients in the University Hospital could be used for teaching purposes, although there were a few private rooms. Those students who were clinical clerks worked very closely with the patients, on assignment and always under supervision. There was a house staff of fifteen physicians at that time, with the dean of the School of Medicine exercising general control. The house staff included Dr. Green Knowlton Dickson, resident in medicine, and Dr. Ralph A. McGill, resident in surgery, with twelve interns in medicine and surgery and one intern in dentistry working under them. Dr. Francis J. Reichman was appointed resident dentist at the University Hospital for the year 1923–24.

There were three separate meetings of each branch of the faculty of the School of Medicine in 1923 and also one joint meeting in the University Hospital on May 4. At a meeting of the Norman branch on January 30, history of medicine was adopted as a new required two-hour course. At the special joint meeting of the Norman and Oklahoma City branches on May 4, in the University Hospital with President Brooks present, the faculty assumed the responsibility of recommending candidates for the degree of Bachelor of Science in medicine.

President Brooks presided at a June 1 faculty meeting in Okla-

[4] *Journal of the Oklahoma State Medical Association*, Vol. XVI (1923), 289.

homa City. Dean Long stressed the responsibility entailed in offering the degree of Bachelor of Science in medicine, which the faculty had recently endorsed. Assuredly, he mentioned the $100,000 appropriation for construction of the building on the Norman campus and asserted that the development of the university during the last decade was a story of vital progress and intellectual uplift. In his opinion this was due in a large measure to President Stratton D. Brooks. At a meeting on August 4 the faculty passed a resolution regretting the departure of President Brooks.

Dr. Buchanan, the acting president of the university, presided at the September 14 meeting. Dean Long regretted that inadequate housing facilities necessitated a denial of admission to the medical school of practically all students applying from outside the state. "The policy of the school," he said, "is to have the entire school under the roof of one medical building. Students of the first two years should mingle with advanced students and should have certain clinical opportunities that will encourage and assist them in their efforts. In that way, the medical student grows into the profession, instead of being abruptly thrown into it after he has spent two years without proper contact with medical matters.

"Among the faculty, there may be those who for one reason or another do not keep up their work regularly. These remarks are not intended for the majority of the members of the faculty, in whose case there is no criticism in this respect, but they are intended for those who accept positions on the faculty and then neglect the essential thing of rendering the expected service."

President Buchanan then made an address of encouragement, stating that the board of regents, as well as the administrators of the university, were wholeheartedly behind the School of Medicine.

There were seventy-eight faculty members of the School of Medicine in the academic year 1923–24. New members added in 1923 were Jacob Martin Essenburg, Ph.D., associate professor of anatomy; Merle Quest Howard, M.D., instructor in neurology; and Joseph Basil Jenkins, D.D.S., instructor in dental surgery. Floyd Jackson Bolend, M.D., associate professor of medicine, was made head of a new hospital Department of Anesthesia in 1923. It was the last year that a course in pharmacy was retained in the curriculum. Kitty Shanklin, a graduate of the University of Oklahoma, was placed in charge of medical social work at the University Hospital.[5]

Twenty-four students graduating from the School of Medicine were granted the M.D. degree in 1923. Among these graduates were George Lumar Borecky, William Edgar Eastland, Herman Fagin, Forrest Merle Lingenfelter, and Phillip Marsden McNeill. During the academic year 1923–24 there were 154 students in the School of Medicine, with admittance denied to practically all applicants outside of Oklahoma because of overcrowded facilities. There were 62 students in the Training School for Nurses, and seven G.N. certificates were granted to the school's 1923 graduating class, including one to Edythe Stith Triplett.

The initial outlook for higher education in Oklahoma during the early part of 1923 was anything but favorable. However, Governor Trapp was able to recreate an atmosphere of confidence, and the legislature came up with several constructive efforts. By passage of the important act that provided for medical and surgical treatment of indigent children at the University Hospital, the stage was set for the construction of a separate children's hospital in Oklahoma City five years later. The legislature also provided funds to build a School of Medicine building. Unfortunately the site selected was on the Norman campus of the university, a decision which was unquestionably influenced by Norman business interests in an attempt to retain all aspects of the university there. This led to a delay in the complete centralization of the School of Medicine in Oklahoma City. However, due to the continued efforts of Dean Long and members of the faculty, a more adequate building for the school was built in Oklahoma City in 1928, and thereby the basis for the University Medical Center was firmly established.

President Stratton D. Brooks was very helpful to the medical

[5] After developing the social service department, Kitty Shanklin (later Mrs. Charles R. Roundtree) became director of the same function at the Children's Hospital of the School of Medicine. She was the first social service worker with the Oklahoma Society for Crippled Children. Subsequently she devoted great energy to various important alumni and university affairs and was awarded a Distinguished Service Citation by the University of Oklahoma in 1961.

faculty during this, his last year at the university. Indeed, his continued interest in the School of Medicine was marked by extraordinarily faithful participation in its faculty meetings, which he attended regularly. His record in this respect was never equalled by his successors.

During 1924, Dr. Carl Puckett became state commissioner of health. He was immediately faced with serious public health problems, especially with widespread typhoid fever, malaria, and pellagra. He appointed Dr. Lucille Spire Blachly to the staff of the Oklahoma Department of Public Health with an assignment to develop a program for reducing infant and maternal mortality rates in the state. Both Dr. Puckett and Dr. Blachly later joined the faculty of the School of Medicine.

The new building on the Norman campus was occupied in February, 1925. All those medical school courses still taught by the College of Arts and Sciences were then transferred to the departments of the School of Medicine housed in the new building. The anatomy department was finally removed from the old wooden structure which it had occupied "temporarily" since 1900.

In Oklahoma City, whose population was approximately 120,000, there were still only the two university buildings, the leased Emergency Hospital and the University Hospital. Paul Fesler continued as superintendent of the University Hospital and chief clerk of the School of Medicine. The 1924–25 catalog and several succeeding ones gave the bed capacity of the University Hospital as 300 beds, but in a report to Dr. Zapffe, Dean Long said it had a capacity of 286 beds in 1924, with 2,888 new patients and 26,661 outpatient visits. Appropriations for the University Hospital were $313,000 for 1924–25, with $1,050,000 for the university.

About this time a new private hospital was developing in Oklahoma City. In 1924, Drs. James E. Harbison and Paul E. Haskett established the Baptist Hospital at 501 N.W. Twelfth Street. The name was changed to Oklahoma City General Hospital in 1927, at which time it had ninety beds and ten bassinets. In 1949 ownership changed again, and it became Mercy Hospital.

There were three meetings of the faculty of the School of Medicine during 1924. At the March 25 meeting, Dean Long presided, and the library committee reported improvements in library service and new regulations for library use. Dr. Turley announced that the School of Medicine was taking over the teaching of physiological chemistry, formerly taught by the Arts and Sciences College.

A resolution was passed urging that the School of Medicine be united in one building on the Oklahoma City campus, adjacent to the University Hospital: "The present geographical division of the school is unfortunate in many respects. There is such a thing as a medical atmosphere, and those who live and move in such an atmosphere, develop an enthusiasm and acquire more readily the information which medical students should acquire."

This faculty resolution went on to emphasize that several years previously the Council on Medical Education had recommended similar action in its survey: "The Association of American Medical Colleges has taken a definite stand in favor of clinical teaching during the first two years. Realizing the necessity of carrying out the plans agreed upon by medical educators in connection with the teaching of medicine and believing that the future progress, if not the life, of this school depends in large part upon uniting the school, [the faculty] appeals to the President of the University and to the Regents to take such steps as may be necessary to bring about the desired union." The resolution was signed by Drs. LeRoy Long and E. S. Ferguson.

Dean Long, presiding at the May 30 meeting, stated, "The better schools of medicine are now making provision for clinical contact not only in the second but in the first year, to provide correlation of the various subjects of the medical course. The problems of the physician present themselves as units and he will solve them only to the extent that he is able to draw on the integrated total of his training. Isolated, uncorrelated information will be of little assistance to him, he cannot use it."

The dean made a comment that the full-time members of the faculty of the School of Medicine were rendering services for inadequate remuneration, mostly because they were willing to work under disadvantages for the present in order to contribute their part to the upbuilding of the institution. A motion was passed that a B minus grade be required for admission to the School of Medicine. A resolution was authorized commending the fine services rendered by Dr. J. S. Hartford, recently deceased. At the meeting on September 10, Dr. Turley reported progress on the construction of the new building for the School of Medicine at Norman.

The small Norman library of the school was given a boost in 1924 by a special additional budget allotted to provide books and periodicals for the newly established Department of Biochemistry and Pharmacology. When the library moved into the new building, a full-time librarian, Agnes Jameson, was employed.

The regents of the university ordered that the university would charge nonresident students in the School of Medicine a tuition fee of two hundred dollars a year, beginning in September, 1924, and that no applicant with less than a B-minus grade average in his premedical requirements should be admitted to the school.

During the academic year 1924–25, there were eighty-five faculty members in the School of Medicine. The following members were added in 1924: Mark Reuben Everett, Ph.D., professor of physiological chemistry and pharmacology; Francis James Warner, M.D., associate professor of anatomy; Homer Lafayette Bryant, M.A., assistant professor of physiology; William Hotchkiss Bailey, M.D., instructor in clinical pathology; James Burnette Eskridge, Jr., M.D., instructor in medicine; LeRoy Downing Long, M.D., instructor in surgery; Joseph C. MacDonald, M.D., instructor in otology, rhinology, and laryngology; Leo Joseph Starry, M.D., instructor in surgery; Wallace Bernard Hamby, B.S., assistant in histology; Ada Reitz Crocker, G.N., superintendent of nurses; and Ruth (Ruby W.) Poindexter, G.N., instructor in nursing.

A new Department of Biochemistry and Pharmacology was established in 1924, with Professor Mark R. Everett as head. The inclusion of these two subjects into one new department terminated several decades of teaching these subjects to medical students by the chemistry department and the School of Pharmacy. In the same year Dr. H. Coulter Todd became professor and head of a separate Department of Otology, Rhinology, and Laryngology, and Dr. E. S. Ferguson became professor and head of the ophthalmology department. Dr. John Frederick Kuhn, Sr. became professor of gynecology.

The 1924–25 catalog of the university states, "Only preliminary work in furtherance of graduate medical instruction for physicians has yet been done in this state."[6] By contrast, graduate courses in the basic sciences had been conducted by members of the medical faculty since 1909, at which time the graduate school of the university was organized. That year graduate courses in anatomy, bacteriology, histology, pathology, physiological chemistry, and physiology were offered. Two years later the anatomy department withdrew from graduate teaching until 1925. In 1924 graduate courses in bacteriology, biochemistry, embryology, histology, pathology, and physiology were offered, but physiology was the only course accredited as a major. In 1925 pharmacology courses were added, the anatomy department resumed graduate teaching, and major graduate courses were offered by all of the basic science departments. The first M.S. degree in basic science subjects was granted in 1921 to Julia Elizabeth Steele in pathology, but it was thirty-four years later that the first Ph.D. degrees were awarded in the basic science subjects.

During the 1924–25 academic year there were 170 students enrolled in the School of Medicine and 45 students in the Training School for Nurses. Twenty-one graduates of the medical school received the M.D. degree in 1924, among whom were Charles Palmer Bondurant and Stanley Francis Wildman. Eleven of the nursing school graduates received G.N. diplomas at the two commencements on June 3 and July 29. Included in this group were Katherine Flemming and Ruby Wadsworth Poindexter. In 1924 Alpha Epsilon Iota, a local professional society for women medical students, was established.

6 University of Oklahoma Catalog, 1924–25, 274.

In 1925 the tenth legislature appropriated $186,000 (House Bill No. 277) for the construction of another new School of Medicine building in Oklahoma City. During February of this same year the first building, constructed at Norman, had been occupied. The 1924–25 catalog did not mention that the $186,000 appropriation for the School of Medicine building was made contingent on the board of regents securing at least an equal amount of matching monies from other sources.

At a meeting of the faculty on June 8, 1925, Dean Long announced that the school authorities were required to raise this equivalent amount of money. He expressed the opinion that the great majority of medical schools, including most of the older schools, favored part-time teachers who, like the ones at the University of Oklahoma School of Medicine, received little or no remuneration for their services. Out of the total income of $189,220 for the School of Medicine in 1925, only $14,000 was paid as fees to the staff of clinical teachers. The dean received a $3,600 salary; full-time professors, $3,800 to $4,500; and assistant professors, $2,200 to $3,800 a year. The University of Oklahoma catalog for 1925–26 showed support for the university in the amount of $1,352,650, exclusive of the $304,000 for the University Hospital and $10,000 for a well for the Oklahoma City campus.

Dr. William Bennett Bizzell, Ph.D., L.L.D., D.C.L., succeeded Dr. Buchanan as president of the University of Oklahoma on July 1, 1925. Dr. Buchanan accepted the post of vice-president. President Bizzell presided at a meeting of the faculty of the School of Medicine for the first time on September 10. Dean Long reported that the new building at the Norman campus had been sufficiently well equipped so that the work of the basic science years could be done with greater facility and accuracy. A resident in pathology had been added to the house organization of the University Hospital. The dean mentioned also that Professor Everett had been asked to supervise the work in biochemistry at the hospital, his status being that of consulting biochemist. In closing the meeting Dean Long again emphasized that the chief end of medical teaching was to instill sound principles that would serve as a sure foundation for the individual who was preparing himself for the important service that he, as a physician, would be called on to render.

At four meetings of the Norman division of the faculty of the School of Medicine in 1925, the following actions were taken: on June 8, a special course in biochemistry was approved for study during the summer school; on September 17, Professor Everett made a preliminary report concerning the committee on honors courses and faculty seminars; and on September 25, a course in pharmacological methods was approved and adopted. The report of the honors committee to establish honors courses at the school was given and adopted subsequently at the October 12 meeting. Supervision of the honors courses was delegated to a committee of three faculty members. The combined Oklahoma City and Norman branches of the library of the School of Medicine were reported to the Association of American Medical Colleges as having 4,500 books, 1,830 bound volumes of journals, and 149 journal subscriptions.

There were eighty-eight members of the faculty of the School of Medicine in 1925–26. Those who had been added during 1925 were as follows: Thomas Mark MacDonald, M.S., assistant professor of pathology; James Robert Reed, B.S., assistant professor of anatomy; Harold Adam Shoemaker, Ph.C., M.S., assistant professor of biochemistry and pharmacology; Green Knowlton Dickson, M.D., instructor in medicine; Bernice Follansbee, G.N., instructor in pediatric nursing; Ada Hawkins, G.N., instructor in nursing; Forrest Merle Lingenfelter, M.D., instructor in obstetrics; Ellis Moore, M.D., instructor in medicine; Flora Weber, G.N., instructor in nursing education and assistant superintendent of nurses; Carl Puckett, M.D., special lecturer in public health and sanitation; J. M. Allgood, assistant in anatomy; and Harry Wilkins, assistant in anatomy.

In 1925, Raymond Lester Murdoch, M.D., become the chief of the outpatient staff, succeeding Dr. Cyril Clymer; Henry H. Turner, M.D., was appointed instructor in medicine. Dr. Turner had come

195

to Oklahoma in October, 1924, as acting medical superintendent of the University Hospital while Dr. Wann Langston was on leave of absence in Europe.

During the same year in which Dr. Turner was appointed to the faculty the Oklahoma State Medical Association took leadership in establishing the first formal postgraduate medical courses available to physicians in Oklahoma. The Commonwealth Fund of New York City and the Oklahoma State Health Department provided financial aid for this undertaking.[7]

The postgraduate program was organized by Luther Wesley Kibler, M.A., on a circuit plan. The program was managed by the University of Oklahoma Extension Division, with the dean of the School of Medicine acting as chairman of an advisory committee. Courses were held at seven different cities in the state under the direction of Wayne Arthur Rupe, M.D., of St. Louis, as instructor in graduate medicine.

The 1925–26 University of Oklahoma catalog contains the following: "*Graduate medical instruction*: While many of the leading physicians of the state feel that they must take at least a few weeks off for study each year, the majority are so situated that this is very difficult or impossible. It has been found in other states that it is entirely practical to bring the instructor to the physician. Graduate medical instruction was begun in the fall of 1925 and the first class . . . met March 1, 1926. One hundred and thirty physicians were enrolled."[8]

Among the twenty-nine graduates of the School of Medicine who received the M.D. degree in 1925 were Donald W. Branham, Leo F. Cailey, Grady S. Matthews, Charles R. Rayburn, and John Harrison Robinson. Certificates of G.N. were granted to twenty-six nurses that year. Sixty-two students were enrolled in the Training School for Nurses, and 177 students were enrolled in the School of Medicine during the academic year 1925–26.

---

[7] Dr. Turner became a member of the Oklahoma State Medical Association's Committee on Postgraduate Teaching in 1932 and its chairman in 1935.

[8] University of Oklahoma Catalog, 1925–26, 311.

The American Hospital Association surveyed the University Hospital in 1926. The association recommended that the dean of the School of Medicine be relieved of direct hospital administration and that a resident physician should be appointed in each clinical department in the hospital. The University Hospital had three hundred beds at the time, according to the 1926–27 university catalog. The Emergency Hospital continued to be used for certain outpatient clinics. According to the *Bulletin of the School of Medicine* for October, 1926, St. Anthony Hospital continued to serve as an affiliated teaching hospital.

Dean E. P. Lyon, of the University of Minnesota School of Medicine, asked permission, in October, 1926, to approach Paul Fesler with an offer to become the superintendent of the University of Minnesota Hospital. Mr. Fesler accepted the invitation, to be effective a year later since he had assumed the additional obligation, in 1926, of the presidency of the Oklahoma State Hospital Association.

Mr. Fesler made an interesting report concerning the method of allocating funds to the University Hospital and the School of Medicine. It was evident that a policy had developed during the five preceding years to allocate those funds used strictly for medical education from the University of Oklahoma budget, while those to be used for the operation of the University Hospital were appropriated separately by the legislature. Thus, the university catalog for 1926–27 reported the sum of $1,418,465 as support for the university exclusive of the University Hospital, which sum included the $186,000 that had been voted for the new School of Medicine building in Oklahoma City. The University Hospital received $304,000, plus a deficiency appropriation of $41,000, according to the 1925 and 1927 Sessions Laws.

The basis for this policy was that the University of Oklahoma, and other state-supported colleges, did not wish to see part of the state's educational funds diverted to the field of medical care. This provides an excellent illustration of political adaptation, since higher education administrators happily deluded themselves into thinking that money was thereby saved for education, but the legislatures merely diverted the necessary funds to the University Hospital before making the appropriations for the University and state colleges. This custom lasted for many years and it finally included the appropriations for the entire medical center.

In spite of the increasing need for a children's hospital in Oklahoma City, Dean Long and Paul Fesler agreed that the construction of a School of Medicine building had top priority and that satisfactory provision must be made for this project by matching the $186,000 appropriation of the legislature. Mr. Fesler also felt that there was a real need for the construction of a private pavilion for the hospital staff at University Hospital. He believed that this construction might be made possible through public contributions, since no state funds were available. Fesler pointed out that the state law required that each county in the state pay fifteen dollars a week for the care of each of its indigent patients at the University Hospital, but that the county commissioners of Oklahoma county had been unwilling to comply with the law.

The Department of Biochemistry and Pharmacology of the School of Medicine was barely two years old when the *Journal of the Oklahoma State Medical Association* ran an interesting editorial entitled "University of Oklahoma School of Medicine Course in Biochemistry and Pharmacology." "None of the medical sciences have made as great and as important advance in recent years as has biochemistry. . . . the average practitioner does not use modern biochemical diagnostic methods to any extent but is content to use older . . . qualitative tests of urine, blood and gastric analysis. On the other hand, hospitals are utilizing modern methods and, having found them valuable aids to diagnosis and treatment, are spending considerable time and effort in keeping their methods up to date. . . . it is encouraging to note that an ever increasing number of physicians and clinics are beginning to use the simpler methods which are indispensable in the scientific treatment of diabetes, nephritis, etc. . . . at least if the physician be acquainted with these analytical methods he can in times of special need do his own analyses or if he gives his work to some commercial laboratory, he becomes a better judge of the results, better able to interpret results and so they are of more important value to him. . . . In this connection it may be of interest to note that the University Medical School has instituted a course of study for physicians and hospital technicians under the direction of the Department of Biochemistry and Pharmacology at Norman."[9]

The young postgraduate teaching program was also expanding during the second year after its organization by Luther Kibler. In the 1926–27 University of Oklahoma catalog it is noted that two additional instructors, Dr. L. D. Thompson and Dr. David Jasper Underwood, had been obtained for the internal medicine circuit course and that a new pediatrics circuit course was being conducted by Dr. W. A. Rupe. There was a total enrollment of 525 physicians in the postgraduate program during the second year.

The House of Delegates of the Oklahoma State Medical Association adopted the following resolution in regard to the postgraduate teaching program: "That this association go on record endorsing the efforts of the University of Oklahoma in its program of postgraduate medical courses offered to doctors of Oklahoma which is a joint program between the School of Medicine and the Extension Department . . . that based upon the high standard of instruction and the type of courses already given, and now being given in several Oklahoma cities, this association recommends to its membership throughout the state that whenever possible they avail themselves of the opportunity for postgraduate study in these courses.

"Further, this association recommends that the various County Medical Societies of Oklahoma will do well to call upon the University of Oklahoma and bring these courses to their respective counties for the benefit of their membership. Resolution adopted."[10]

Further comment followed to the effect that some physicians had traveled regularly from forty to seventy-five miles each week to attend the lectures and that the success of the program had exceeded all expectations. The officials of the extension department

9 *Journal of the Oklahoma State Medical Association*, Vol. XIX (1926), 110.
10 *Ibid.*, 234.

of the university were so impressed with the response and enthusiasm of the physicians of the state that they promised a course would eventually be offered in every county having fifteen or more doctors. "Provided that able instructors can be secured, the School of Medicine is planning to offer other subjects through the Extension Division next year. The future of the work, and its expansion, also depends to a great extent upon the appropriation of funds to assist in bearing the administrative expense now being carried by the division."

President Bizzell presided at a meeting of the faculty on June 5, 1926, when Dean Long reported that the school had not been able to secure the money to supplement the capital appropriation of the last legislature. Then he mentioned that there was some objection to the present medical graduates as being unwilling to locate in rural districts because their training was such that it made them averse to locating in rural areas. The dean believed that this was not the result of present medical training but rather that it was because good roads and automobiles made it possible for patients in the rural communities to be transported readily to hospitals in towns or cities, leaving a country physician with but little to do outside of emergencies. "The physician of the rural community is not supported," the dean said. "This is a serious matter and we should render whatever service we may be able to render to improve the situation."

At this same faculty meeting President Bizzell called attention to the growing need for both a dental school and a program of public health education.

The minutes of the Norman branch of the faculty of the School of Medicine show that on April 27, 1926, approval was given to consolidate materia medica and pharmacology into one course to be known as pharmacology II. Also, a motion was passed that during the next academic year all students be required to pass general examinations in all subjects of the first two years of medicine at the end of the second semester of the second year.

On May 31, the honors committee recommended to the faculty that Robert H. Akin and Mable Eckstedt Hart be granted the honor

200

recognition of magna cum laude for special work in bacteriology and biochemistry, respectively. The faculty voted approval of the recommendation and also that Samuel H. Alexander be granted similar recognition of cum laude for his achievement as an outstanding student with the highest general average for the first two years. At a September 21 meeting rules governing the management of the animal house were adopted.

There were ninety-five faculty members of the School of Medicine during the academic year 1926–27. The following new faculty members were appointed: William Alfred Buice, B.S., assistant professor of bacteriology and hygiene; Wendal Doop Smith, M.S., assistant professor of histology and embryology; Edith Brewer, G.N., instructor in obstetrical nursing; James Jackson Caviness, M.D., instructor in ophthalmology and otorhinolaryngology; Warren Troutman Mayfield, M.D., instructor in physical diagnosis; Earl Duwain McBride, M. D., instructor in orthopedic surgery; Phillip Marsden McNeill, M.D., instructor in medicine; Grider Penick, M.D., instructor in gynecology and instructor in surgery; Thirza Powell, instructor in nursing; Edith Ruth Tilton, B.S., instructor in dietetics; Ralph Edward Chase, B.S., assistant in physiology; and Fay Sheppard, M.S., assistant in biochemistry and pharmacology.

In the October 15, 1926 – March 17, 1927 issues of the *University of Oklahoma Bulletin of the School of Medicine* is the following formal statement: "Honors to be conferred at the commencement at which the student receives the degree of Bachelor of Science in Medicine, including a general honor, cum laude, a special honor, magna cum laude, or in the case of highest excellence, summa cum laude, for those students who pass a special examination in modern languages, do extra work in some department of the preclinical years, carry on certain lines of investigation, and present an acceptable thesis." Detailed requirements of the program are given in these bulletins.

The tuition fee for nonresident students at the School of Medicine in 1926 was one hundred dollars a semester. University approval was given to the recommendations of the Norman branch of the faculty of the School of Medicine by a statement in the 1926–27 university catalog that students completing the second year of study in the School of Medicine were required to pass a general examination in all subjects and courses of the first two years before advancement to the clinical years.

During the academic year 1926–27 there were 182 medical students and 87 nursing students in training at the university. Forty medical graduates were granted the M.D. degree in 1926. Included in this number were Herbert Dale Collins, George Henry Kimball, Ivo Amazon Nelson, John Copeland Pickard, Fenton Almer Sanger, and Mallalieu McCullagh Wickham. Among the fifteen nursing graduates receiving G.N. certificates was Edith Brewer.

The 1925–26 biennium witnessed the arrival of Dr. William Bennett Bizzell from Texas as the sixth president of the University of Oklahoma, a position he was to retain until 1941. He found the School of Medicine building on the Norman campus newly occupied and funds appropriated by the tenth legislature to duplicate it on the Oklahoma City campus. Because of a matching requirement this action did not lead to immediate construction, but it signified that the legislature had made a most important and correct decision as to the unification of the School of Medicine. The launching of the postgraduate program for physicians and the honors research course for medical students were other progressive steps.

It is interesting that in 1926 Dean Long mentioned the public complaints of too few medical graduates locating their practices in rural districts of the state. He attributed this maldistribution to the preference of citizens in small communities to be transported by automobile over good roads to the larger towns and cities. However this situation has persisted for decades and was not cured by any of a variety of special attempts to influence young physicians. Indeed, the problem is far more complicated than Dr. Long believed. It has no simple answer for it is part of the trend to urbanization. The graduates of the University of Oklahoma School of Medicine have maintained an enlightened attitude in regard to the problem.

202

XI. The Hospital for Crippled Children and the Unification of the School of Medicine: 1927–28

HENRY S. JOHNSTON, of Perry, defeated O. A. Cargill, mayor of Oklahoma City, for the office of governor of the state of Oklahoma in the 1926 election. Johnston had been a leader in the Constitutional Convention in 1906, and was a member of the State Senate, serving as president pro tempore.

The eleventh legislature began its session in January, 1927, under the leadership of D. A. Stovall as speaker of the house and of Mac Q. Williamson as president pro tempore of the senate. Governor Johnston was able to work in reasonable harmony with the legislative body at first and was helpful in accomplishing the enactment of several bills of considerable importance to the University of Oklahoma School of Medicine. He delivered a special message to the legislature, requesting that a hospital for crippled children be built in Oklahoma City and placed under the direction of the University Hospital authorities. Subsequently, Senate Bill No. 75,[1] authorizing the State Board of Affairs to build and equip such a hospital in connection with and under the University Hospital, to be known as the Oklahoma Hospital for Crippled Children, was approved on February 18, 1927. The bill provided that the cost of the hospital was not to exceed $300,000, the actual amount appropriated.

A second act of major significance, Senate Joint Resolution No. 3, stated that because it had been impossible for the regents of the university to secure from other sources the matching funds required

[1] *Session Laws,* 1927, Chapter 19, 20.

for the $186,000 appropriated by House Bill No. 277 in 1925, for the purpose of constructing a new School of Medicine building in Oklahoma City, the senate and the house of representatives were directing the board of regents to let a contract not to exceed $250,000, to finance the construction of such a building at the University Hospital. A further sum of $64,000 was being appropriated for the year ending June 30, 1928. This resolution was approved on March 9, 1927. The 1926–27 and 1927–28 catalogs of the University of Oklahoma state correctly the sums given above for the two construction projects.[2]

A third involved piece of legislation, House Bill No. 170, entitled "Medical and Surgical Treatment of Children," amending a 1923 act, was also approved on March 9, 1927.[3] In this bill the age limit of the indigent child was raised and defined as "any person under the age of 21 years afflicted with some malady that can be cured or remedied." County judges were authorized to commit, with the parents' consent, any such indigent child to the University Hospital and the Hospital for Crippled Children and to assign plastic and orthopedic cases to other approved hospitals in the state. Through a one-tenth mill levy the bill created a separate, county Crippled Children's Fund but its effectiveness was limited by a decision of the state supreme court which denied the right of the University Hospital to levy charges against the counties.[4]

House Bill No. 170 also established free general clinics for children to be held in each congressional district in Oklahoma as a duty of the School of Medicine faculty. The faculty was also assigned the responsibility of establishing standards for the clinics. To qualify for participation under this law area physicians and hospitals had to make application to the dean of the University of

[2] An erroneous figure of $350,000 for the Hospital for Crippled Children was given in two sources, see Gittinger, *The University of Oklahoma*, 134, and Edward Everett Dale and Maurice L. Wardell, *History of Oklahoma* (New York, Prentice-Hall, 1948), 347.

[3] *Session Laws*, 1927, Chapter 81, 122.

[4] *Oklahoma Reports*: Cases Determined in the Supreme Court, Vol. CXXII, No. 17411, February 15, 1927, 268. "The Supreme Court rules that the State University Hospital may not enter into contracts with counties or municipalities and force them to pay for their patients."

Oklahoma School of Medicine and be officially approved by the medical faculty. In addition the bill provided that the faculty could approve plastic and orthopedic specialists on its own initiative.

Lew Wentz, an oil man and philanthropist of Ponca City, Oklahoma, was very interested in the care of children at the University Hospital, and he made a great effort to secure the passage of the crippled children's hospital acts. For two entire months he was in almost daily attendance at the state Capitol on behalf of both Senate Bill No. 75 and House Bill No. 170, which were eventually passed with only one dissenting vote.

According to Dr. Basil Hayes, Mr. Wentz had at one time proposed making a donation of $300,000 to build a suitable children's hospital for the teaching staff of the School of Medicine, a sum which the legislature had agreed to accept and supplement by furnishing the grounds and the equipment. However, the author has not been able to find confirmation of this statement.

To place Mr. Wentz's activities in proper historic perspective, it should be recalled here that Earle R. Bridges, president of the Oklahoma City Rotary Club, had proposed that a statewide Society for Crippled Children be organized. Lewis Haines Wentz was invited to attend the organizational meeting on September 24, 1925. Bridges became the society's first president, and Mr. Wentz, a charter member, was the first treasurer. Joe Hamilton, principal of the Ponca City public schools, accepted the post of permanent secretary. His salary was donated by Mr. Wentz over a period of many years.[5]

An outstanding effort of the Society for Crippled Children, from 1926 to 1936, was the conducting and financing of the diagnostic Crippled Children's Clinics, in which about ten thousand children around the state were examined during the ten-year period. The Oklahoma Commission for Crippled Children shared this work and the expense, starting in February, 1936.

Lew Wentz was born in 1881 in Mt. Vernon, Iowa. He came to

[5] In addition to the material in Dr. Earl D. McBride's article "The Oklahoma Society for Crippled Children," *Chronicles of Oklahoma*, Vol. XXVII No. 2 (1949), the author is indebted to H. Dick Clarke, executive secretary of the Oklahoma Society for Crippled Children, for further information relative to the society and Lew Wentz.

Ponca City in 1911, was taken into the Oklahoma Hall of Fame in 1942, and died in 1949. During his lifetime he was recognized nationally as an outstanding leader in the crippled children movement in America. Cora Miley, writing in *Harlow's Weekly* in 1932, said that Lew Wentz, a millionaire philanthropist, was the most popular man in Oklahoma and that he was so well liked because of his simplicity, generosity, modesty, and sincerity.

Concerning the University of Oklahoma, the eleventh legislature also modified the law creating the board of regents by requiring that at least three members of the board be alumni of the university and by providing that members could be removed only through impeachment proceedings.

In 1927 the board of regents approved free medical care for a period of two weeks for faculty members of the School of Medicine and for hospital employees and student nurses. The regents also approved a 20 per cent discount for state officials, state employees, and University of Oklahoma faculty members, employees, students, physicians, graduate nurses, and ministers.

The Council on Medical Education and Hospitals had reduced the number of schools of medicine to eighty by 1927, of which sixty-two were class A schools with four-year curricula and nine were class A with two-year curricula. There were three class B and six class C schools. That same year the council began to approve residency programs in hospitals.

The University Hospital appropriations for 1927–28 were, as now customary, separate from those of the university.[6] The main hospital received $215,000 in salaries and $140,000 in maintenance, while the Hospital for Crippled Children was allotted $18,940 in salaries and $54,750 in maintenance, a total of $428,690.

According to the 1927–28 university catalog the support for the university was $1,377,500, aside from its allocations for construction of the new buildings.

The same catalog stated that the first- and second-year medical courses would be transferred from Norman to Oklahoma City in

6 *Session Laws*, 1927, Chapter 90, 139.

206

September, 1928, and that all instruction in the School of Medicine would then be concentrated in Oklahoma City, where the new medical school building was under construction at the corner of Phillips and N.E. Thirteenth streets and the Hospital for Crippled Children was going up at the corner of Kelley and N.E. Thirteenth streets.

In the midst of all this activity in 1927, Paul Fesler left the University of Oklahoma to become superintendent of hospitals at the University of Minnesota. To say that the State University Hospital and School of Medicine experienced a severe loss is an understatement, for Mr. Fesler had labored incessantly for the improvement of the whole institution. He had traveled Oklahoma from border to border, contacting legislators, physicians, and all others who could possibly be interested in the growth of the School of Medicine. It goes without saying that his assistance to Dean Long had been of incalculable value.

The faculty of the School of Medicine met on June 2, 1927, with President Bizzell present and Dr. Long presiding. Dr. Long expressed the opinion that all concerned with the approaching consolidation of the medical school in Oklahoma City were very happy about the whole prospect. President Bizzell said he was pleased to report that there was now a kindlier feeling between the university and those citizens in Norman who had opposed the complete transfer of the School of Medicine to Oklahoma City. Dean Long emphasized that the merging of interests on one campus would be accompanied by greater burdens on the teaching staffs because of the expanding demand on the clinical services as soon as the new Hospital for Crippled Children was opened.

Dr. Long realized the necessity for strengthening clinical departments, but just how this was to be done was still debatable. He did feel very strongly that the clinical teacher was a better teacher for having practiced his profession and a better doctor for having taught. In other words, he preferred the part-time clinical teacher.

Dr. Everett made a report to the faculty on the requirements for the honors degree. He stated that a student receiving this degree must be in the upper fourth of his class, must pass a reading examination in modern French or German, and must submit a thesis of research work on some original topic, in addition to the pursuit of the required medical studies.

A second faculty meeting, at which Dean Long presided, was called on December 2 to submit the names of the committee for carrying out the provisions of the recently passed crippled children's law. Drs. George A. LaMotte, Samuel R. Cunningham, Abraham Blesh, and Robert M. Howard were named to this committee.

At an April 28 meeting of the Norman branch of the faculty of the School of Medicine a committee was appointed by Assistant Dean Turley to take charge of the general examinations to be given to second-year students. The committee consisted of Dean Turley, Dr. Ellison, and Dr. Everett. On October 4, 1927, Assistant Dean Turley reported that construction had started on the new building for the School of Medicine in Oklahoma City.

There were ninety-four members of the faculty in 1927–28. Appointed in 1927 were: Hugh Gilbert Jeter, M.D., assistant professor of clinical pathology; William Arthur Meyers, M.D., assistant professor of biochemistry and pharmacology; and George Lumar Borecky, M.D., instructor in genitourinary diseases. Dr. Don Horatio O'Donoghue, M.D., was appointed resident in orthopedic surgery. During the year the faculty started a new bimonthly publication of original papers, entitled the *Bulletin of the University School of Medicine.*

Concerning postgraduate courses, the 1927–28 general catalog reported that during the year circuit courses in internal medicine were given by Dr. D. J. Underwood, and a short course in physiotherapy was offered by Dr. F. B. Granger. Dr. Alice Wild Tallant gave two lecture series on obstetrics at a number of centers, and other short courses of one week each were offered at the School of Medicine in surgical diagnosis, internal medicine, and tuberculosis diagnosis and treatment. It was stated in the catalog that the extension division had enjoyed the hearty co-operation of the State Board of Health through its Bureau of Maternity and Infancy.

There were 815 physicians enrolled in the graduate medical courses during the year ending June 30, 1928.

The catalog for the year reported 188 medical students enrolled in the School of Medicine, but there was no separate listing of nursing students for the same period. Forty-two graduating medical students received the M.D. degree in 1927. Among these were August Malone Brewer, Fanny Lou Brittain, Brunel DeBost Faris, Hervey Adolf Foerster, Henry Washington Harris, Gilbert Lewis Hyroop, William Arthur Meyers, Nesbitt Ludson Miller, Clifford W. Moore, James Robert Reed, Harry Wilkins, and John Powers Wolff. Nineteen graduates of the School of Nursing received G.N. certificates in 1927. The title, director of the school of nursing, was used in this and succeeding catalogs, having been first conferred on Ada Crocker.

A report of the Committee on Medical Education of the Oklahoma State Medical Association in 1928 stated that the medical department of the university was just completing a building on the Oklahoma City campus of the School of Medicine which would be ready for occupancy at the beginning of the next term. Through its increased facilities the school's classes could be enlarged. The report also called attention to the early completion of a new hospital for children on the campus, increasing the number of beds under direct control of the School of Medicine to over four hundred. "It is the definite plan of all concerned," the report concluded, "to create a great medical center in connection with the School of Medicine at Oklahoma City—a center that will offer technical and clinical opportunities to the physicians of the state—and we call attention to these facilities and opportunities in the hope that the physicians of the state will take advantage of them."[7]

The construction of these facilities was the first step in the building of a consolidated medical center on the Oklahoma City campus of the University of Oklahoma. The opening of these facilities on August 1 and September 1, 1928, were red-letter days in the history of the School of Medicine. Offices, laboratories, the

[7] *Journal of the Oklahoma State Medical Association*, Vol. XXI (1928), 159.

library, and other functions of the school were moved from the Norman campus and from the Emergency Hospital (Oklahoma General Hospital) to the new School of Medicine building, 801 N.E. Thirteenth Street, on August 1. Classes for medical students were transferred there in time for the full utilization of the new facility on September 1. The building was of classical architecture, a four-story, fireproof structure, 190 feet long and 80 feet wide, containing 54,670 square feet of floor space, with lecture rooms, laboratories, a library, museum, and offices for the staff of the School of Medicine.[8] Facilities for research, as well as those for instruction in the medical sciences, were provided, including an animal house on the roof of the building. The 1928–29 *Bulletin of the School of Medicine* referred to the old Emergency Hospital on Third and Stiles streets as the Clinical Building, since it was being used for certain outpatient clinics.

The new Crippled Children's Hospital was also completed during the year, at N.E. Thirteenth Street and Kelley Avenue. It was a three-story fireproof building with a capacity of 160 beds. The total cost of this building of 76,263 square feet was approximately $414,000, a further appropriation having been made for this purpose in 1929. This hospital, like the main University Hospital, was under the administration of the regents of the University of Oklahoma.

On November 1, 1928, the alumni of the School of Medicine gathered in Oklahoma City and devoted a full day to clinical meetings. The joint dedication of the School of Medicine and the Hospital for Crippled Children took place the following day. The principal speaker at the dedication of the School of Medicine building in the forenoon was Dr. Jabez N. Jackson, former president of the American Medical Association, who discussed the value of a medical education. John Rogers spoke on "The Medical School from the Regent's Standpoint," and Doctor Long delivered an address on the "Ideals of the Medical Profession." The University of Oklahoma Glee Club concluded the morning program with

8 University of Oklahoma catalog, 1927–28, 47.

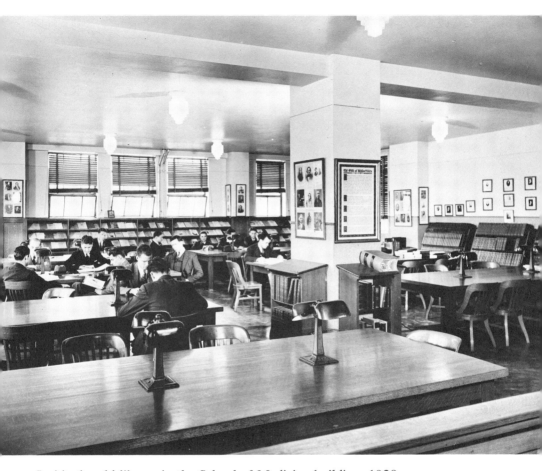

Inside the old library in the School of Medicine building, 1928.

Courtesy University of Oklahoma Medical Center

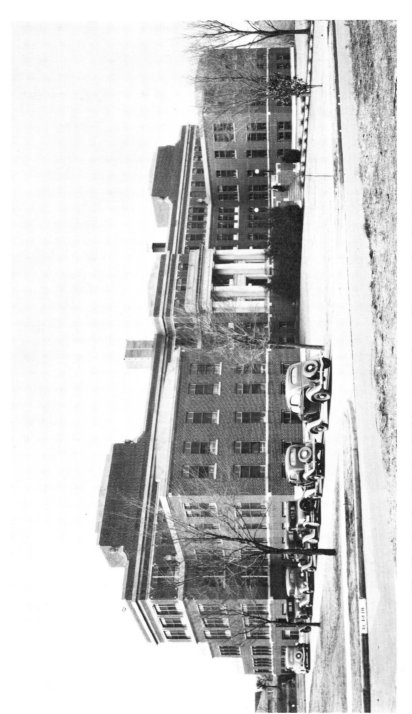

The Hospital for Crippled Children in Oklahoma City, completed in 1928.

Courtesy Sooner Medic

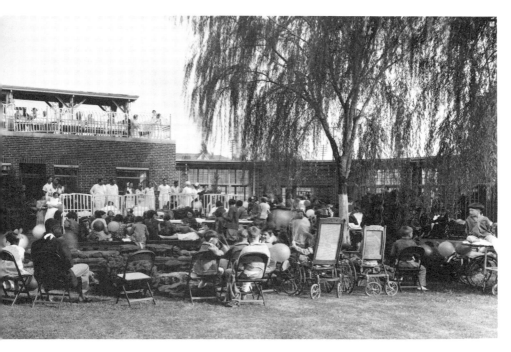

An outdoor program for patients at the Hospital for Crippled Children.

Courtesy University of Oklahoma Medical Center

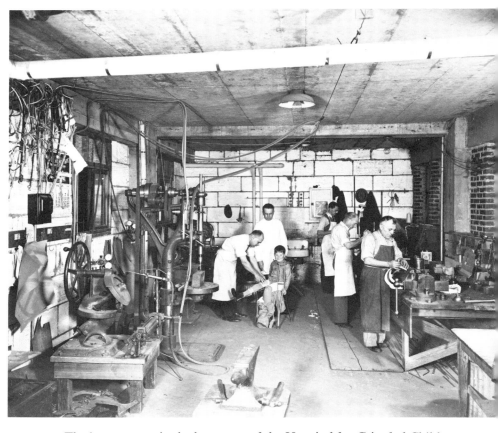

The brace room, in the basement of the Hospital for Crippled Children.

Courtesy University of Oklahoma Medical Center

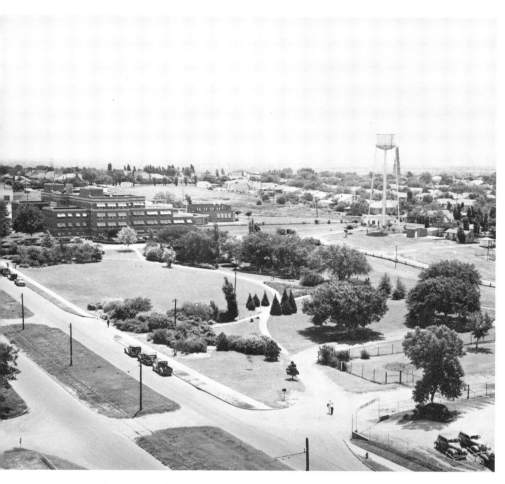

The University of Oklahoma Medical Center in Oklahoma City, 1928.

Courtesy University of Oklahoma Medical Center

215

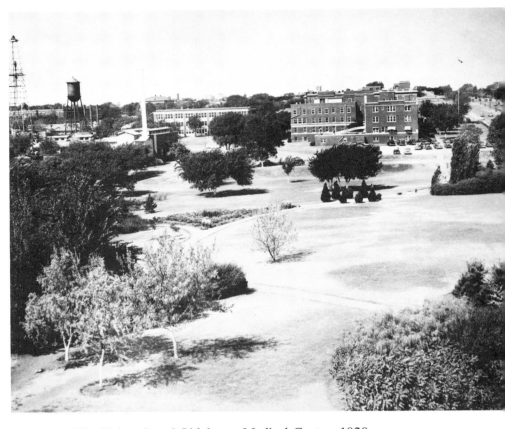

The University of Oklahoma Medical Center, 1928.

Courtesy University of Oklahoma Medical Center

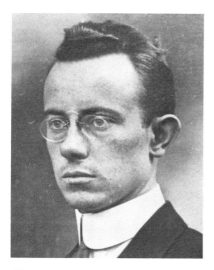

Curt Otto Von Wedel, Jr., M.D., director of the outpatient staff, 1911–12.

Courtesy Oklahoma State Board of Medical Examiners

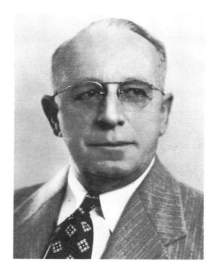

Cyril E. Clymer, M.D., director of the outpatient staff, 1917–24.

Courtesy Oklahoma City Academy of Medicine

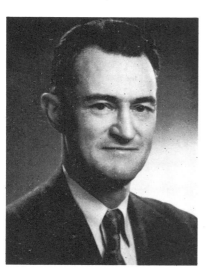

Raymond L. Murdoch, M.D., director of the outpatient staff, 1925–31.

Courtesy Oklahoma City Academy of Medicine

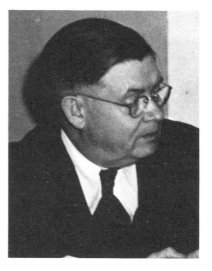

Paul H. Fesler, acting superintendent of university hospitals, 1916–18; superintendent of university hospitals, 1918–20; and fiscal superintendent of university hospitals, 1920–27.

Courtesy University of Oklahoma Medical Center

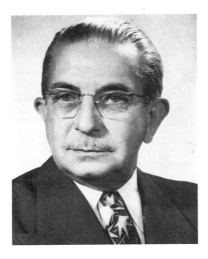

Henry H. Turner, M.D., acting medical superintendent of university hospitals, 1924–25.

Courtesy Oklahoma City Academy of Medicine

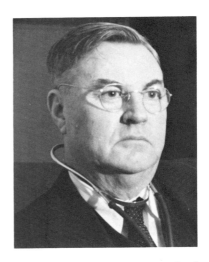

Wann Langston, M.D., medical superintendent of university hospitals, 1920–27; superintendent of university hospitals, 1927–31; and director of the outpatient staff, 1931–33.

Courtesy Sooner Medic

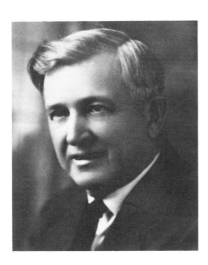

John Bodle Smith, M.D., superintendent of university hospitals, 1931–33.

Courtesy Dr. W. K. Haynie

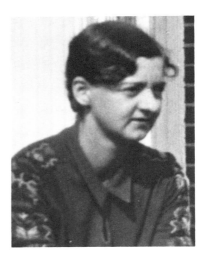

Edith Ruth Tilton, director of the dietetic intern program, 1928–32.

Courtesy Mrs. Mary Zahasky

musical selections. At the afternoon dedication of the Hospital for Crippled Children the principal speaker was Governor Henry Johnston. His address emphasized the appeal of the crippled child to the public and the high ideals of the medical profession.

In an October 16, 1928, letter to Dr. Long, former Governor R. L. Williams, then judge of the United States District Court, wrote that he could not attend, saying, ". . . . You know how I looked forward during my administration to such an accomplishment. When I became governor in 1915 the School of Medicine was housed in a rented frame building and it was classed by the American Medical Association as a B class institution. . . . It was then that I planned to get an appropriation to build a hospital owned by the state and to be operated by the state, so that the school could be in the A class. It was with that view that you were selected as dean to bring about that progress in medical education in this state, and I congratulate you upon the great work you have done. It is a vindication of my constructive planning and foresight and I shall look back to the University Hospital and everything that is on that ground as a result of my administration, and one of the achievements of it, and you can readily understand how I regret not being present. I remember the opposition that we encountered from private hospitals. My response was that the University Hospital in place of injuring private hospitals would aid them; that we would establish a center of medical learning and of clinics in this state that would attract from other states. Please indicate on that occasion my regret at not being able to be present."

There was enthusiastic public approval of the new Hospital for Crippled Children. In an October 30, 1928, telegram Edgar F. "Daddy" Allen, secretary of the International Society for Crippled Children, expressed to Dean Long the hope that "the key to the doors of the Crippled Children's Hospital, which you dedicate on November 2, may be lost—to the end that the doors will always be open for the reception of little children." Perhaps one of the most vigorous expressions was incorporated in a newsletter of the Oklahoma Society for Crippled Children, affirming an earlier tribute

219

which appeared in the *Daily Oklahoman.* "The Crippled Children's Hospital is one of the few Christly things that stand out on Oklahoma's ledger."[9]

Charles F. Long stated in his article "With Optimism For The Morrow" that one of President Bizzell's major accomplishments was the development of the University Medical Center with his support of the initial request for $750,000 to build the Hospital for Crippled Children and the Medical School building on the Oklahoma City campus. The author quoted President Bizzell as saying, "There have been many marvelous moments. One of the greatest was the time Governor Johnston signed the bills authorizing the erection of the Medical School building and the Crippled Children's Hospital, and at the same instant Lew Wentz handed me a check for $50,000 to add to the Lew Wentz loan fund."[10]

The completion of these two buildings and the consolidation of all the medical instruction on the Oklahoma City campus was a great triumph for Dr. LeRoy Long, who by this time had become well known throughout the country. The following excerpts are from the address given by Dean Long at the dedication of the School of Medicine building. "A little over ten years ago we were doing the best we could in temporary quarters at Norman and in wholly inadequate rented property here at Oklahoma City [before the Main University Hospital building was erected]. . . . Then we had another dream—a dream with a vision—the vision of a building here on the campus of the School of Medicine which would house the entire school, and now that dream is a reality. . . . During the developmental period of an institution there is only one way by which success can be achieved and that is through the complete loyalty and cooperation of the faculty. . . . we now have a faculty of almost 100 and they have stood as they stand now in an unbroken phalanx in support of the administrative officers of the School. . . . but even with a loyal faculty and money to build houses and buy equipment we could not succeed without the great central

9 *Newsletter,* Oklahoma Society for Crippled Children, No. 3 (February, 1965), 40.

10 Long, "With Optimism for the Morrow," *Sooner Magazine,* Vol. XXXVIII (September, 1965), 34–35.

support of the University with its wise President and Board of Regents, . . . and now that we are entirely off the principal campus I feel the necessity of keeping in close and intimate touch with the University with a keenness that I never realized before. Without our connection with the University we could not exist as a respectable Medical School. . . .

"I have already referred to the assistance that the school has received from the medical profession, but I cannot permit this opportunity to pass without emphasizing our gratitude to the physicians of the state. I have every reason to believe that the School has their active support, and I regard that support as one of our most important assets. No class of citizens is better able to intelligently judge the work of the school, because they are able to accurately appraise the product of our efforts in both the training of students and the treatment of patients in our hospitals and clinics. . . . In this solemn hour I pledge the best efforts of this faculty to maintain our ideal, and to see to it that the work done in this house shall be useful to the people of the state."[11]

The medical profession's viewpoint on medical education in 1928 should not be overlooked. It may best be illustrated by some quotations from an address by Dr. Arthur Dean Bevan, chairman of the Council on Medical Education and Hospitals. "The question of uneven distribution [of physicians] will be solved, as far as it can be solved, by the economic, social, climatic and other influences which control the lives of men, but it will of course to a certain extent always remain with us. It certainly would not be influenced in any way by training a poor grade of physicians. . . . Medical education cannot be left safely in the hands of the medical profession alone. . . . but it is very evident that the medical school cannot be safely left in the hands of the universities alone; something more is needed. Uprooted from the medical profession, uprooted from the community, and transplanted to the scientifically prepared soil of the university campus the medical school will lack those things which the medical profession and the community alone can give. . . . We must not permit a line of cleavage, a schism, to

11 *Journal of the Oklahoma State Medical Association*, Vol. XXII (1929), 65.

221

develop between the medical profession and the medical teachers in our university schools of medicine. . . . We must not allow our universities to build and conduct hospitals for the primary purpose of teaching medicine. We must bring about a situation wherein the communities will build and conduct hospitals for the proper care of the sick, and the best of these will be used as teaching hospitals. No hospital should ever be built unless its primary purpose and function is to care for the sick. . . . The medical educator who sees the future of medical education as a purely university affair, with its clinical teaching conducted at a university owned hospital heavily endowed and filled only with charity patients and officered by full time salaried men, with a hospital with its patients and the laboratory with its frogs and guinea pigs, conducted along the same scientific university ideal lines, without any contact with the medical profession and the community, surely has no vision and no place in the future development of medical education in this country."[12]

In 1928 the Council on Medical Education and Hospitals discontinued its classification of medical colleges as A, B, and C schools.

Another progressive step on the Oklahoma City campus in 1928 was the construction of a Crippled Children's School building as an adjunct to the new Hospital for Crippled Children and a very generous replacement of the one small room made available for this function in the University Hospital in 1925. This facility, known as Lew Wentz Hall, was a gift from Lew Wentz, of Ponca City, which he undertook after making a tour of inspection of hospital schools in various parts of the United States with President Bizzell and an architect. The 3,430 square foot, $37,230 building was constructed at a cost of only $18,230 because, according to the records in the Oklahoma Society for Crippled Children, friends of Mr. Wentz contributed most of the building materials.

When occupied in January, 1929, this building was one of the most attractive and well-equipped hospital schools in the nation. There were two large classrooms, an auditorium, and an office. It

[12] *Journal of the American Medical Association*, Vol. XC (1928), 1173.

was connected with the Crippled Children's Hospital by long corridors lined with large French windows and enclosing a beautifully landscaped court where the children could enjoy the sun. A library of well-chosen books was installed and managed by the Oklahoma Hospitality Club. Motion picture films were shown weekly by the Moving Picture Machine Operators Union. Grace B. Smith, who started to work in the school when it opened, became its principal.

In the 1928–1929 university *Bulletin of the School of Medicine* St. Anthony Hospital was mentioned as an affiliated teaching hospital with a two-hundred-bed capacity. There were eighteen hundred beds at the Central Oklahoma State Hospital in Norman, another affiliate. The population of Oklahoma City at that time was approximately 150,000.

The University of Oklahoma 1928–29 catalog and the Session Laws of 1927 showed the following state support for the two university hospitals: the University Hospital, $215,000 in salaries and $140,000 in maintenance; the Crippled Children's Hospital, $37,880 in salaries and $109,500 in maintenance, making a total of $502,380. The support for the university that year was $1,507,500. There was a supplementary appropriation for the School of Medicine of approximately $59,340 to provide salaries for several additional faculty members, to move equipment from Norman to Oklahoma City, and to pay for the installation of utilities, equipment, and furniture in the new School of Medicine building. Most of the furniture was fabricated at the state penitentiary.

Selection of interns and residents was made by a board known as the Hospital Committee. This group represented all of the larger clinical departments and it set the policies of medical administration for the hospitals. Some of the outpatient clinics were still conducted in the old Emergency Hospital building at Third and Stiles streets, since the outpatient department was not removed totally from it until 1929–30. During 1928 there were 4,425 patients in the main University Hospital alone.

All meetings of the faculty of the School of Medicine in 1928 were held prior to the dedications of the two new buildings. The branch of the faculty at Norman met on May 10, and formed a committee to conduct the general examination; its last separate meeting was held May 28, 1928, when honors degrees were awarded to Alvin W. Lehew and Gordon G. Bulla. Dr. Thuringer was appointed chairman of the Library Committee of the School of Medicine.

Dean Long presided at a June 1 general faculty meeting when he commented that the School of Medicine had just completed its last year as a school divided geographically and that, for the first time in the faculty's history, it could start out as a unit. Inasmuch as there would be approximately four hundred hospital beds with combined facilities under direct control of the faculty, he felt that there would be a need for some full-time clinical personnel to develop fully the opportunities for proper teaching and clinical research that would become available. Constant supervision of certain laborious details connected with outpatient service and clinical instruction on the hospital wards was an obvious necessity in the dean's opinion. Stating that it was time to re-examine the curriculum of the School of Medicine, Dean Long appointed a curriculum committee consisting of Dr. W. Langston, chairman, Dr. L. A. Turley, and Dr. L. J. Moorman.

At the September 14 meeting Dean Long presided again, with President Bizzell present. The dean greeted the faculty by saying, "When we take into consideration the efforts and aspirations of the University authorities and the faculty of the School of Medicine during the last 13 years, I am sure that the opportunity of meeting in this new building for the School of Medicine gives all of us a great deal of pleasure. We have passed one more milestone and a very important one." He proposed the creation of committees on graduate courses and fellowships. Dr. Langston then made a report for the curriculum committee which was approved by the faculty. He indicated that the fourth-year students had been given a much larger service in the outpatient department than formerly. The committee believed that the third-year student should work in the hospital and the fourth-year student should work in the outpatient clinics, insofar as the clerkships were concerned. New courses on allergy and physical therapy were added. Dean Gittinger, Emil R.

Kraettli, and George E. Wadsack, from Norman, attended this meeting.

There were 110 members of the faculty of the School of Medicine in 1928–29. Members newly appointed in 1928 included the following: Vaclav Kuchar, M.D., professor of physical therapy; Edward Charles Mason, M.D., Ph.D., professor of physiology; Mabel E. Smith, M.A., associate professor of nursing education and director of the School of Nursing; Myron Thomas Townsend, Ph.D., associate professor of histology and embryology; Edith T. Aitken, director of internships in dietetics; Margery Ardrey, B.S., instructor in dietotherapy; Clarence Edgar Bates, M.D., instructor in medicine; James Garfield Binkley, M.D., instructor in obstetrics; Charles Palmer Bondurant, M.D., instructor in dermatology; Caroline T. Burnet, G.N., instructor in practical nursing; Herbert Dale Collins, M.D., instructor in gynecology; William Edgar Eastland, M.D., instructor in dermatology; Norphleete Price Eley, M.D., instructor in medicine; Verna Foster, G.N., instructor in theoretical nursing; Frederick Redding Hood, Ph.C., instructor in biochemistry and pharmacology; Ruth Evelyn Hoppock, A.B., instructor in elementary dietetics; Cecil Willard Lemon, B.S., instructor in physiology; James Patton McGee, M.D., instructor in ophthalmology; Lawrence Chester McHenry, M.D., instructor in otology, rhinology, and laryngology; James Floyd Moorman, M.D., instructor in medicine; Don Horatio O'Donoghue, M.D., instructor in orthopedic surgery; Frances J. Reichmann, D.D.S., instructor in dental surgery; and James Byron Snow, M.D., instructor in medicine. Green Knowlton Dickson, who had left the faculty in 1926, returned and was reappointed as instructor in medicine in 1928.

The following excerpt is from the 1928 report of the Committee on Medical Education of the Oklahoma State Medical Association, "We wish to call attention to the work in medicine by the extension division of the State University. Already groups of physicians in all parts of the state have taken part in these extension courses, and it is our information that the service had been appreciated by the profession generally. . . . There are frequent conferences between the Dean of the Extension Division of the University and a committee composed of members of the faculty of the School of Medicine, and it is through these conferences that the final plan of procedure is decided and the proposed instructors approved."[13]

The 1928–29 university catalog mentions a requirement of a reading knowledge of French or German or six college hours of either one for entrance to the School of Medicine. The *Bulletin for the School of Medicine* for the same year states that "a reading knowledge of German or French is strongly urged."

Up to the time of the occupancy of the new library quarters in the Medical School building on the Norman campus in 1924, there had been no full-time librarian for the school. Agnes Jameson was the first person to occupy this position, as far as available records indicate. The exact date of her appointment is not known, but she served as librarian until her part-time assistant, Grace Swain (later Mrs. John McCarty Cassidy) became librarian in 1927. Mrs. Cassidy served until her husband graduated from the School of Medicine in 1931. In 1928 the combined book stock at Oklahoma City was 4,025 volumes.[14]

The internship in dietetics at the University of Oklahoma School of Medicine and hospitals was organized about 1928. It was approved by the American Dietetic Association that same year. The B.S. degree in home economics was required for entrance, and a certificate was given on completion of the one-year internship course. One dietetic student, Winifred Reynolds McGowan Dailey, completed this program in 1928.

There were 199 medical students and 115 nursing students enrolled during 1928–29. Forty-one of the graduates from the School of Medicine received M.D. degrees in 1928. Included were Robert Howe Akin, John Milton Allgood, James Franklin Campbell, Louis H. Charney, Darrell Gordon Duncan, Floyd Gray, Wallace Bernard Hamby, Patrick Sarsfield Nagel, and Robert Leonard Noell. Fifteen nursing students, including Ada Hawkins, received G.N. certificates.

13 *Journal of the Oklahoma State Medical Association*, Vol. XXI (1928), 159.

14 Some of this information was obtained from a typewritten manuscript entitled "The University of Oklahoma Medical School Library Handbook," which is in the files of the library of the School of Medicine.

The biennium ending in 1928 was one of triumphant achievement for Dean Long and the School of Medicine. In 1927 the eleventh legislature passed bills to erect the Hospital for Crippled Children on the School of Medicine campus in Oklahoma City and a new School of Medicine building, funded without any provisos for matching money. Certain citizens of Norman who had protested the moving of the complete medical school to Oklahoma City were now willing to abandon their antagonism.

The legislature also passed a bill for the medical and surgical care of children at the Hospital for Crippled Children which, as soon as erected, became a center for many statewide aspects of the medical care of children. This bill also established support for free clinics for children throughout the state and authorized the appointment of eligible plastic and orthopedic surgeons and other hospitals in the state to participate in the program. These functions both required approval by the faculty of the School of Medicine.

Beneficial community efforts in respect to the medical care of children appeared throughout the state, and the groups concerned co-operated very well with the School of Medicine and the university hospitals. The most active organization of this nature was the Oklahoma Society for Crippled Children, formed in 1925. Lew Wentz, the philanthropist from Ponca City, offered to help in these efforts because of his experiences with the society. Indeed, he was undoubtedly the single most effective agent in securing passage of the bills mentioned. Thus, the university hospitals created firm ties with the public in a fashion that would have been difficult to achieve by other parts of the university. The faculty of the School of Medicine believed very definitely that it had important duties in connection with community needs. Joe Hamilton should also be mentioned as the very capable and inspired man who stemmed out of the Society for Crippled Children and who guided state health affairs concerning children over a period of years.

There were also other happenings in this period. The new legislative act concerning the regents of the university rendered their appointment inviolate except by impeachment. A dietetic internship was organized in 1928. Also at this time the University Hospital lost the services of Paul Fesler, who had been a great help to Dean Long.[15]

When the new buildings had been completed, the departments, courses, and equipment were transferred from the School of Medicine building at Norman to the new building on the Oklahoma City campus. This was a notable step forward because it created the basis for the future university medical center, although official designation of the University of Oklahoma Medical Center as such did not occur until twenty-eight years later. Centralization of the school and the hospitals in Oklahoma City led to an immediate expansion of medical training, an increase in the number of medical students, and the first effective facilities for medical research available to the faculty of the School of Medicine. The joint dedication of these buildings on November 2, 1928, therefore, marked the beginning of a new epoch. Medical education itself was maturing throughout the country as well as in Oklahoma, increasing the need for greater co-operation between practitioners and teachers of medicine. The medical school was soon in need of a few full-time clinical professors, a fact which Dean Long acknowledged but hesitated to remedy. The well-known town and gown syndrome was developing!

15 It is of special interest that Oklahoma legislators commended Paul Fesler for his valuable services to the state. See, *Session Laws*, 1927, Chapter 272.

XII. Innovation and Fulfillment: 1929–30

MEMBERS OF THE TWELFTH legislature gradually became very critical of Governor Johnston and demanded that his secretary, who was the object of violent legislative criticism, be discharged, alleging that she had far too much influence over the governor's actions and policies. On March 20, the senate voted thirty-five to nine to impeach the governor. It sustained a single charge—incompetency, thus acquitting Governor Johnston of all other charges. As a consequence, William Judson Holloway became the eighth governor of Oklahoma on March 20, 1929, just as the financial depression started to sweep through the nation.

Governor Holloway had come to Oklahoma from Arkansas, where he was born in Arkadelphia in 1888. He had been principal of the Hugo High School before receiving his law degree at Cumberland University. He was elected to the state senate, where he served as president pro tempore. Governor Holloway was a friend of the teaching profession and a popular governor for the most part, but there was some purely political criticism of his appointment of Lew Wentz, a Republican, as chairman of the State Highway Commission. During his administration the State Historical Society Building was constructed.

The twelfth legislature appropriated an additional $150,000 for the completion and equipping of the Oklahoma Hospital for Crippled Children by passing House Bill No. 4, which was signed into law by Governor Holloway.[1]

1 *Session Laws*, 1929, Chapter 70, 88.

The 1929–30 university catalog was the first university catalog to report a medical center type of budget in which all appropriations to the School of Medicine, the School of Nursing, and the university hospitals were budgeted separately from those for the remainder of the university. The catalog gave the appropriated funds for the Oklahoma City campus as follows: to the School of Medicine, salaries, $82,000, maintenance, $48,520, land purchase, $22,500, making a total of $153,020; to the State University Hospital, salaries, $220,000, maintenance, $136,000, totaling $356,000; and to the Crippled Children's Hospital, salaries, $79,-250, maintenance, $100,000, totaling $179,250. The full appropriation for the Oklahoma City campus amounted to $688,770. The operational support for the Norman campus of the university at the time was $1,515,636 ($1,764,136, including buildings and repairs).

The catalog also stated that the outpatient department of the School of Medicine was not in the "Clinical Building," but now was located in the State University Hospital and the Children's Hospital. The facilities and arrangements for outpatient work in these hospitals were described as very good, with separate quarters for the various departments and with 100–150 patients being treated daily. Judging from a letter of July 23, 1930, from Dr. Wann Langston to a member of the board of regents, the outpatient clinic was probably removed from the "Clinical Building" at Third and Stiles streets in the fall of 1929; this building was still designated by that name in the *Bulletin of the School of Medicine* on October 15, 1929.

The 1929–30 catalog credited the University Hospital with 225 beds, whereas a contemporaneous article in the *Journal of the Oklahoma State Medical Association* stated that there were 275 beds in that hospital and that an additional 100 beds would be available when the Hospital for Crippled Children was completed.[2]

2 *Journal of the Oklahoma State Medical Association*, Vol. XXII (1929), 93. Reports by the Council on Medical Education and Hospitals on hospitals approved for internship indicate that 386 beds were available during 1929–30, as contrasted with 275 in the 1927–28 biennium.

There were only twenty private rooms in all at the university hospitals in 1929. St. Anthony Hospital had 200 beds at the time.

Dean Long terminated the position of assistant dean that year, creating a new appointment of administrative officer of the School of Medicine and the university hospitals. Dr. Wann Langston filled this position from 1929 to 1931. Dr. Long also made use of an executive or advisory committee composed of five to seven faculty members.

Dean Long presided at four meetings of the faculty between January 18 and April 23, 1929. At these meetings a report of the committee on summer school was approved. A motion was passed that the honors degree be conferred at the time the student finished his full medical course and received his M.D. degree. The honors committee was reappointed, with Dr. Joseph M. Thuringer, chairman, and Drs. Mark Everett and Edward C. Mason, members. Dr. Thuringer, who was also chairman of the library committee, reported that the Oklahoma County Medical Association had donated its library to the School of Medicine. The curriculum committee made a recommendation that the school require a fifth or hospital year before issuing the diploma of Doctor of Medicine, to become effective with the graduating class of 1933. This motion passed, and the October, 1929, *Bulletin of the University of Oklahoma School of Medicine* carried the announcement that "Beginning with the class of 1933 the M.D. degree will be withheld until satisfactory completion of a year's general internship served in an accredited hospital." This requirement was later withdrawn.

At a fifth faculty meeting on September 16, President Bizzell presided, since Dean Long was absent from the city. At this meeting the faculty adopted a recommendation by the curriculum committee that a supervised library hour be instituted for first- and second-year students.

There were 121 members of the faculty at the Oklahoma City campus in 1929–30. Newly appointed in 1929 were the following: William Paul Newell Canavan, Ph.D., associate professor of bacteriology; Candice Lee Monfort, G.N., associate professor of nursing education and director of the School of Nursing; David Thomas

Bowden, M.D., assistant professor of epidemiology and public health; Frank Lester Else, B.S., assistant professor of physiology; Carmen Russell Salsbury, M.D., assistant professor of anatomy; Ida Lucile Brown, B.S., instructor in bacteriology; Leo F. Cailey, M.D., instructor in otology, rhinology, and laryngology; James Franklin Campbell, M.D., instructor in anatomy; Karl La Von Dickens, M.S., instructor in anatomy; Margaret Fitzgerald, G.N., instructor in surgical technique; Katherine Fleming, G.N., instructor in nursing education and superintendent of the Hospital for Crippled Children; Ephraim Goldfain, M.D., instructor in neurology; Rufus Quitman Goodwin, M.D., instructor in medicine and director of clinical clerkships; Wilhelmina Hinnenkamp, G.N., instructor in operating room technique; Florence Ingram, G.N., instructor in obstetrical nursing; Mary Ella Jones, G.N., instructor in principles and practice of nursing; Joseph Willard Kelso, M.D., instructor in gynecology; Wendell McLean Long, M.D., instructor in gynecology; Julia Martin, G.N., instructor in theoretical nursing; Floriene Ann Mueller, G.N., instructor in pediatric nursing; Charles Ralph Rayburn, M.D., instructor in neurology; Charles Ross Rountree, M.D., instructor in orthopedic surgery; and Edythe Stith Triplett, G.N., instructor in nursing education and assistant director of the School of Nursing. Dr. Ward Shaffer was the resident dentist at the University Hospital in 1929.

The 1929–30 catalog of the university stated that a reading knowledge or ten college hours of French or German (or six college hours if the subject was also taken in high school) was required for entrance into the School of Medicine. Elective courses were offered in the curriculum of the School of Medicine for the first time in 1929, as noted in this catalog. There were 288 total hours of such courses.

Medical and surgical clerkships in the School of Medicine, as part of the curriculum for the third and fourth years, were first listed in its 1929–30 bulletin published in October, 1929. Rufus Q. Goodwin of the Department of Medicine was in charge of these clinical student clerkships.

In an article in the *Journal of the Association of American*

Medical Colleges, Dr. Goodwin outlined the purpose and operation of these clerkships, as presented originally by him at the annual meeting of the Association of American Medical Colleges in Rochester and Minneapolis on October 30, 1933. Dr. Goodwin mentioned that Dr. Fred C. Zapffe had formulated definite clinical clerkships at Northwestern University School of Medicine in 1927, the first instance of clinical clerkships in this country being supervised by one man. He told how the clinical clerkship for fourth-year students at the University of Oklahoma School of Medicine was revised in 1929, and, through the efforts of Dr. Wann Langston, a clinical clerkship course was placed in the third-year curriculum also. It provided for one and a half hours of daily instruction by a supervisor. Dr. Goodwin devoted half time to this course.[3]

One of the early objectives of the clerkships was to carry the preclinical study into the clinical aspects of medicine. Dr. Goodwin quoted Dean Lyon of the University of Minnesota School of Medicine as saying in 1929: "I followed a master of diagnosis in his day's work. I saw him elicit reflexes and measure temperatures; I heard him speak of valves and pressure and enzymes and neurons and calories. I said, 'that man is not practicing medicine he is practicing physiology.' I watched a therapeutist at the bedside and found that he was not practicing medicine but pharmacology. I saw a surgeon earning $1,000; I discovered that he was not practicing surgery but anatomy, pathology, physiology and high finance. Finally, the relation I was seeking came suddenly into mental view. Anatomy and physiology and pharmacology and bacteriology and all the rest are not the children of medicine; they are not the branches of an evolutionary tree; they are not handmaids; they are not stepping stones or preparatory stages. They are it. They are medicine itself." Similar reasoning led to the inclusion in 1929 of two new courses at the University of Oklahoma School of Medicine, namely, applied biochemistry and clinical physiology. Both courses were given in the third year as joint courses of the Department of Medicine and the two basic science departments.

The 1929–30 university catalog states that honors for medical

3 *Journal of the Association of American Medical Colleges*, Vol. IX (1934), 229.

students would be conferred at the commencement with the degree of Doctor of Medicine and would consist of special citations endorsed by the faculty of the school. Further requirements for these honors were outlined in the description of work. Since the honor program was a method of encouraging original research by medical students, it is interesting that the University of Oklahoma also conferred its first Ph.D. degree in 1929.

In 1929, Luther Kibler received the title of director of postgraduate medical study. The 1929–30 catalog mentions that during the year short extension courses in nose and throat, internal medicine, diagnosis, physical therapy, surgical diagnosis, obstetrics and gynecology, and pediatrics had been offered. A course in children's dentistry was given for the first time, during April and May, 1929, and Dean Arthur C. Black, of Northwestern Dental College in Chicago, and five other members of the faculty gave a six-week course in postgraduate dentistry in five state centers. During 1929 officers of the Oklahoma State Medical Association approached the Extension Division of the University of Oklahoma in regard to a picture film service for county medical societies. The State Medical Association purchased these films and the extension division booked them.

There were a number of comments on the postgraduate work in the *Journal of the Oklahoma State Medical Association* for 1929. A note was included that Muskogee physicians co-operated with the extension department in organizing a course in surgical anatomy and cadaveric surgery, under the direction of Dr. J. C. Stephenson of the University of Oklahoma School of Medicine. An editorial in the association's journal complimented the course given to Muskogee physicians, inasmuch as fourteen physicians secured nine weeks of dissection, surgical anatomy, and cadaveric surgery at a very nominal sum. This was a night course in surgery, so there was very little interference with the routine practice of the doctors.

At the house of delegates meeting of the association on May 27, 1929, Dr. J. M. Byrum, of Shawnee, stated that he desired endorsement by the medical association for an appropriation for the extension work of the university which had been going on for a number of years. A committee was appointed, and it drew up a resolution stating that the medical profession of Oklahoma endorsed the work of the Extension Division of Oklahoma University in providing postgraduate medical courses conducted by nationally recognized specialists throughout the state. It was earnestly recommended that the legislature continue appropriations for this work. The report was adopted unanimously.[4]

There were 223 medical students at the university during the academic year 1929–30. Thirty-eight graduates of the School of Medicine received M.D. degrees in 1929. Among them were Edmund Gordon Ferguson, Euel P. Hathaway, Patrick Henry Lawson, Emil P. Reed, Leroy Huskin Sadler, Delbert G. Smith, O. Alton Watson, and Neil Whitney Woodward.

In the 1929–30 catalog of the University of Oklahoma the School of Nursing was listed separately for the first time, with the following statement: "The courses in the theory and the practice of nursing are given by instructors especially prepared in nursing. Courses are also conducted by members of the faculty of the School of Medicine, and the work of the School in general is under the direction of the School of Medicine. There is now a separate Bulletin by the University for the School of Nursing."

There were 162 students in the School of Nursing during the year 1929–30. Twenty-one graduates of the school in 1929 received certificates of Graduate Nurse. Among these was Josephine Mesley.

William H. Murray returned to Oklahoma in 1929, after an absence of nearly a decade, including a five-year stint at colonization in Bolivia. In 1930 he entered a vigorously contended primary in an effort to secure the nomination for governor. He won,

---

[4] The 1929 postgraduate program exceeded the budget; the Oklahoma State Medical Association gave some financial assistance for several years. For further historical details regarding the postgraduate medical program, see "Editorial," *Journal of the Oklahoma State Medical Association*, Vol. XXVI (1933), 450, and Henry H. Turner, "Postgraduate Medical Education in Oklahoma," *Journal of the Indiana State Medical Association*, (March, 1940), 126.

though he previously had been denied this objective several times since statehood. His innate political sense told him that this was the hour for using his particular variety of politically strategic baiting, a skill he had developed through long experience as a participant in the political life of Indian Territory, at the 1907 Constitutional Convention in Guthrie, where he was the presiding officer, and as a member of the first legislature of Oklahoma. There had been public comment on his arbitrary rulings and seizure of power on more than one occasion. The Farmers' Union, in trying to bring pressure on the makers of the constitution, found a ready contact through William H. Murray. Murray apparently regarded his personal views as always the correct ones, and anyone who opposed him he viewed as the "tool of corporate interests."

Those who can recall the dramatic tumbling of the stock markets in the fall of 1929 and the great financial depression that ensued, can understand how this situation served as a political aid to candidate Murray, since many farmers were debt-ridden and discouraged. He conducted a singular campaign, travelling back and forth across the state in an ancient Model T. Ford. He employed personal invective against his opponent, Frank Buttram, a regent of the University of Oklahoma. Murray designed his speeches for a "plain folks" appeal. It was not long before this method of campaigning began to gain publicity. Thus, "Alfalfa Bill" Murray, the reincarnation of the frontier politician, "reaped the harvest of discontent" and practically coasted into the statehouse as the ninth governor of Oklahoma.

As governor, Murray harassed institutions of higher learning. He hounded them about expenditures, claiming that colleges made "high toned bums" out of students. An editorial in the *Tulsa Tribune* on November 6, 1930, painted a dark picture: "[Murray] has threatened the institutions of higher learning with a 'bomb shell'. He has already destroyed years of effort by the state's educators and the friends of the colleges by coming out in opposition to the constitutional amendment proposing non-political boards of regents for the Agriculture and Mechanical College and the University. . . . Murray is groping blindly in the labyrinth of history.

He is hopelessly confused. . . . Oklahoma is in for four years of governmental instability, reaction and turmoil."

The thirteenth legislature appropriated a total of $668,250 for the fiscal year 1930–31 to the medical school and hospitals of the University of Oklahoma: to the School of Medicine, $82,500 for salaries and $32,500 for maintenance, making a total of $115,000; to the University Hospital, $220,000 for salaries and $150,000 for maintenance, totaling $370,000; and to the Crippled Children's Hospital, $81,250 for salaries and $102,000 for maintenance, a total of $183,250. The support for the Norman campus was $1,630,636.

The total budget for the School of Medicine that year was $134,-570. Dean Long's salary, after fifteen years of devoted service, was finally raised to five thousand dollars. Dr. Wann Langston was still administrative officer, both for the School of Medicine and its hospitals, and Candice Monfort Lee, G.N., was director of the School of Nursing and superintendent of nurses. Harry C. Smith became office manager of the University Hospital on May 1, 1930.

Dr. Bart W. Caldwell, secretary of the American Hospital Association, made a hospital survey for the Chamber of Commerce of Oklahoma City in 1930. His report lauded the University of Oklahoma Medical Center and said that the two university hospitals had few equals in the United States. He reported that Oklahoma City spent less than other cities (less than twenty-five cents per capita) for health and hospitalization of its indigent sick. He urged the city to build a 250-bed city-county hospital near the Medical Center campus. His report showed that the University Hospital and St. Anthony Hospital had about the same number of patients. However, the University Hospital treated 452 Negro patients during the year, and the Oklahoma General Hospital treated 245, as contrasted with fourteen at St. Anthony Hospital.

In 1930, after the outpatient department had been moved to its new quarters in the university-owned hospitals, the social service department function was extended to the Hospital for Crippled Children, and field work was started for students of the University

237

of Oklahoma. Until 1928 the departmental administrative staff at the University Hospital consisted of only the director, one case worker, and one stenographer; that year another case worker and a second stenographer were added at the Children's Hospital. In 1930 the number was raised to a total of seven, by the addition of another worker and stenographer.

There were three meetings of the faculty of the School of Medicine in 1930. President Bizzell was present on January 28 when Dr. Long presided and Dr. Langston reported on the meeting of the Association of American Medical Colleges to which he had been a delegate. The Oklahoma County Medical Society expressed the desire that the School of Medicine aid in organizing an Oklahoma City Clinical Society and asked the dean to appoint a committee for that purpose.[5] The faculty set the minimum requirement for admission to the School of Medicine as an average of C, based on the new rating plan.

At a June 4 meeting a resolution was passed by the faculty in memory of Dr. Antonio D. Young. "We who have worked with him and have been close to him for many years likewise realize his sympathy and kindness and appreciate intensely the loss of one who has been an intimate part of our daily work and lives. He was always considerate of those about him, conservative in his opinions and statements, tolerant of opinions of others and in the words of Emerson . . . 'There is something in the man finer than anything he said—a power to make his talent trusted.'"[6]

On September 19, Dean Long presided at the last faculty meeting of the year. The old but still difficult problem of the scarcity of physicians in the rural districts was discussed once more. The dean announced the appointment of Dr. Fishman as head of the Department of Neurology, with Dr. Langston assuming the responsibility of Dr. Fishman's medical service. Dr. Goldfain was appointed an additional member of the neurology department, and it was an-

---

[5] The fall conferences of the Oklahoma City Clinical Society have been successful annual affairs ever since the society was organized in 1930.

[6] *Journal of the Oklahoma State Medical Association*, Vol. XXIII (1930), 206.

nounced that Dr. Henry Turner would be appointed to some proper position in the department on his return from study abroad.

There were 130 members of the faculty of the School of Medicine in the academic year 1930–31. Those who joined the faculty during the year were as follows: Carl August Nau, M.A., assistant professor of physiology; Gertrude Helen Wilber, M.S., assistant professor of histology and embryology; Robert Howe Akin, M.D., instructor in urology; Fannie Lou Brittain, M.D., instructor in pediatrics; Carl Langley Brundage, M.D., instructor in dermatology; Francis Asbury DeMand, M.D., instructor in obstetrics; Darrell Gordon Duncan, M.D., instructor in dermatology; George Harry Garrison, M.D., instructor in pediatrics; Bert Fletcher Keltz, M.D., instructor in medicine; Walter Archibald Lybrand, J.D., lecturer on medical jurisprudence; Elizabeth McGoldrick, M.A., instructor in psychiatric social work; Josephine Mesley, G.N., instructor in pediatric nursing; John Alfred Moffett, M.D., instructor in anesthesia and head of the department; J. Walker Morledge, M.D., instructor in medicine; Elmer Ray Musick, M.D., instructor in medicine; William Marcus Mussil, M.D., instructor in otorhinolaryngology; Mavis Richbourg, B.S., instructor in nursing education; Glen Alexander Russell, instructor in anatomy; Ward Loren Shaffer, D.D.S., instructor in dentistry; and Mary Whelan, M.S., instructor in biochemistry and pharmacology. Mrs. Grace Swain Cassidy was listed in the 1930–31 catalog as the librarian of the School of Medicine in Oklahoma City. Ernest Freeman Hiser was appointed medical artist for the school.

During the year, pediatrics became a separate department, with Professor William M. Taylor as its head. The Department of Anesthesia was headed by Instructor Moffett and, as mentioned previously, Dr. Fishman was appointed head of neurology. Dr. Charles Lincoln White became head of the dental surgery section in 1930, and Dr. Frank Pitkin Bertram was appointed resident dentist.

The 1930–31 catalog listed 412 hours of total electives during the last three years of the curriculum of the School of Medicine and

239

announced that, beginning with the class of 1933, an internship would be required to qualify for the M.D. degree. "The Medical School feels justified in requiring this fifth year for the issuing of the diploma," was a comment at a house of delegates meeting, May 7, 1930. "That matter has been up for consideration time after time . . . has been unofficially discussed for several years. . . . It is a pretty broad step."[7] As a matter of fact, it never was put into effect at the University of Oklahoma.

In 1930, forty-seven M.D. degrees and thirty-eight certificates of G.N. were awarded. Among those who received the M.D. degree were William Alfred Buice, Fred Redding Hood, Milam Felix McKinney, Bert Ernest Mulvey, E. Cotter Murray, William Gerald Rogers, and Edward T. Shirley. There were 229 students in the School of Medicine and 134 in the School of Nursing during the academic year, 1930–31.

The postgraduate program continued to expand under the able direction of Luther W. Kibler. An appraisal of the postgraduate medical and dental instruction was presented in the 1930–31 catalog of the university: "Physicians and dentists in the State of Oklahoma are now depending upon the State University for their postgraduate studies each year. . . . Many are now coming into the courses who have been unable to pay the high costs of going away to distant research centers for further study. . . . There is first hand evidence of a higher standard of practice and an improvement in public health conditions within the state as a result of these postgraduate courses. Four to six short courses of postgraduate medicine are offered each year at the School of Medicine of the University, with the extension division handling the administrative part of the program. One or two circuit courses, with seven centers in each circuit, are offered in the state each year. One circuit course in postgraduate dentistry is likewise offered in the state. . . . There are in Oklahoma 2,370 physicians and 765 dentists."

An editorial in the 1930 *Journal of the Oklahoma State Medical Association* commented that it was true that many unusual and

7 *Ibid.,* 217.

worthwhile courses were offered to physicians in various parts of the state, but, as might be expected, the greater number of courses were given in Oklahoma City. Several courses in Tulsa and Muskogee were also well attended, at a minimum cost to the physician, with the course in anatomy and cadaveric surgery, at Muskogee, being very helpful.[8]

A letter, addressed to Dr. Leonard C. Williams, president of the Alumni Association of the School of Medicine of the University of Oklahoma, on March 6, 1930, from Dr. N. P. Colwell, secretary of the Council on Medical Education and Hospitals, replied to Dr. Williams as to the qualifications necessary for deans of medical schools. Dr. Colwell emphasized the importance of a dean's awareness of the requirements of a modern medical school and stated that a dean should also be able to administer the affairs of his institution in a manner sufficiently diplomatic to insure that the best work could be accomplished with the least friction. Dr. Colwell informed Dr. Williams that during the past ten to fifteen years, as some medical schools had grown and expanded, arrangements for employment of full-time deans had been made.[9]

Dr. Leonard Williams was evidently the first medical alumni president. He was born in 1897 in Leclede, Idaho. Dr. Williams graduated from the Oklahoma School of Medicine in 1920, and was chairman of arrangements that same year for the celebration of the restoration of the school to a class A rating.[10] It appears that the first alumni association declined in activity after 1935 and that the present reorganized and very active association was formed in 1938.

It was in this biennium that Dean LeRoy Long reached the pinnacle of his achievement, but it was merely a whimsy of fate

8 *Ibid.*, 126.

9 On May 8, 1929, the regents and the president of the university discussed "the situation with reference to the deanship of the Medical School" and "the desirability of a full time Dean beginning with the opening of the fall term in September." At that time it was the opinion of the board of regents that a full-time dean be employed.

10 Dr. Williams stated that an alumni association of the School of Medicine first came into existence in 1930, and he provided a copy of the original constitution of the organization which is on file in the library of the School of Medicine.

that permitted him to witness the full realization of his dream before the anti-intellectual twilight that was to descend in 1931.

Governor Holloway, like his predecessor, had been of assistance to the University of Oklahoma School of Medicine and to the university hospitals on the Oklahoma City campus. In particular Governor Holloway aided the completion of the Hospital for Crippled Children. After its completion the final transfer of all off-campus outpatient activities to the university hospitals marked the termination of School of Medicine activities in rented property. The medical division of the university on the Oklahoma City campus now had 386 hospital beds in use.

The president and regents of the university made a significant improvement by separating the budgets of the schools of medicine and nursing and of the university hospitals from the main budget for the university on the Norman campus. This action was bound to minimize future intra-university contentions over appropriated funds, while at the same time preserving the fiscal authority of the regents.

During 1929–30 the medical faculty was enlarged to 130 members, and 412 hours of elective courses were developed in the medical school curriculum. The faculty of the School of Nursing was also increased substantially, and in 1929 the school began to publish its own bulletin.

Development of medical and surgical clerkships for the School of Medicine in 1929, under Dr. Rufus Q. Goodwin, was a very progressive step in the bedside education of medical students. The postgraduate courses for physicians also continued developing, with innovations during both years of the biennium.

The appropriations for the institutions on the Oklahoma City campus had increased to about two-thirds of a million dollars annually. Dr. Caldwell, secretary of the American Hospital Association, found, on inspection, that the university hospitals now had few equals throughout the country. He noted specifically that they provided medical and surgical care to approximately twice as many Negroes as any other Oklahoma City hospital. The social service

242

activities of the university hospitals doubled with the opening of the Hospital for Crippled Children.

Despite the many favorable accomplishments, a menacing political cloud was gathering strength. Undoubtedly this threat to Dr. LeRoy Long prompted Dr. Williams, the first president of the newly created alumni association of the School of Medicine, to contact the secretary of the Council on Medical Education and Hospitals early in 1930 for advice and suggestions. Dr. Williams' request was dictated by rumors which had come to his attention in regard to the antagonism of William H. Murray toward the dean of the School of Medicine.

XIII.   The End of an Era

THE WHOLE STATE SYSTEM of higher education suffered drastically during the governorship of William H. Murray. As a gubernatorial candidate he assailed higher education in a bid for votes, denouncing the University of Oklahoma as an antagonist of agriculture. He promised to throw a bomb into the state's educational system if elected, and, once he had achieved his goal, he proceeded to make good his promise. Governor Murray falsely accused William Bennett Bizzell, president of the University of Oklahoma, of inadequacy as an educational leader and of permissiveness as a mentor and monitor, charging mismanagement of funds by the administrative personnel and immorality and drunkenness among the faculty.

The Board of Regents of the University of Oklahoma, in executive session on March 7, 1931, took under consideration the various charges leveled at the administration, as well as similar charges against several members of the faculty at Norman. The board passed a resolution requesting the legislature to make a thorough investigation of all the charges that had been reported in the newspapers. On one occasion the governor dispatched a special agent to Norman to investigate "flagrant immorality and corruption." He continued this vendetta by sending the Oklahoma National Guard to collect tickets at a football game, claiming that the ticket monies were mismanaged.

The senate approved a resolution on February 3, authorizing an investigation of the Student Union Building Corporation at the

244

University of Oklahoma.[1] On March 28, at the request of the regents, the senate approved a second resolution, empowering a senate committee "to make a thorough and complete investigation of charges of immorality and corruption at the University of Oklahoma in Norman; whereas certain newspapers recently have stated that an investigation made at the University of Oklahoma by Alva McDonald has revealed the existence of immorality and unlawful expenditure of state funds."[2]

In the manner of a demagogue, the governor circulated his personal propagandizing organ—a weekly folio-type paper known as the *Blue Valley Farmer*, which carried large advertisements from the university and other state colleges. Evidently Governor Murray saw no conflict of interest in this use of state funds.

It is small wonder that by June President Bizzell had become concerned about rumors that Governor Murray had designs to remove him from his position as president of the University of Oklahoma. Presidents and faculty members of other colleges in the state became fearful for their positions, too. Their fears were justified, for Governor Murray succeeded in replacing more educators than any former Oklahoma governor, with the exception of Jack Walton.

During Governor Murray's 1931 "firebells campaign" his secretary sent a letter to President Bizzell urging "voluntary" campaign contributions of at least two dollars from each faculty member. This was only one of the actions which led to national criticism of the governor's educational policies by such publications as the *New Republic*. The May 18, 1932, issue of the *New Republic* stated, "He ['Alfalfa Bill' Murray] is an incorrigible enemy of academic freedom. Since he has been Governor he has instituted what is little less than a reign of terror among the publicly supported educational institutions of the state. His motto is that any educator who draws his pay from the state treasury must be for Alfalfa Bill, first, last and always. . . . Like the famous Bilbo of Mississippi, Governor Murray has never heard of freedom of

1 *Session Laws*, 1931, Senate Resolution No. 5, 378.
2 *Ibid.*, 380.

speech in the classroom, wouldn't understand it if he did hear of it, and obviously would not respect it even if he ever discovered what it is all about."

Murray appointees constituted a majority of the regents of the University of Oklahoma by May, 1931. During the year, Governor Murray appointed William J. Milburn, of Sayre, to succeed Mrs. Addie Lee Lowther, of Guthrie; Raymond A. Tolbert, of Oklahoma City, to succeed Frank Buttram, of Oklahoma City; Judge Claude C. Hatchett, of Durant, to replace Breck Moss, of Oklahoma City, whose appointment by Governor Holloway had not been confirmed by the senate; and Malcolm E. Rosser, Jr., of Muskogee, to succeed John Rogers, of Tulsa. He reappointed George L. Bowman, of Kingfisher, who then became the new president of the board, replacing Frank Buttram. Other regents who remained on the board were John A. Carlock, of Ardmore, and Joe C. Looney, of Wewoka.

Governor Murray did not reserve his vitriolic and slanderous assaults for college presidents and their faculties alone. On the contrary, as soon as he became governor, he promptly removed his "enemy number one," Lew Wentz, from the chairmanship of the State Highway Commission. The following year the governor issued one of his numerous executive orders, arbitrarily ousting Lew Wentz from the commission entirely. He was thwarted in this abortive attempt, however, by the state supreme court, which overruled the governor's action. Murray probably had the last laugh anyway, because in 1933 the fourteenth legislature co-operated by creating a totally new highway commission! It should be stated for the record that Mr. Wentz donated to the Oklahoma Society for Crippled Children, his favorite philanthropy, whatever monetary reward he realized from his position on the highway commission.

Governor Murray's second enemy appears to have been Dean Long and the University Hospital. As early as January 30, 1931, we have record of a letter to Dean Long from Dr. John A. Haynie, of Durant, regarding "an intimation in today's Daily Oklahoman that Dr. Long might be removed as dean." Even earlier there was a letter of January 15, addressed to President Bizzell, in which Dr. Wann Langston tendered his resignation as administrative officer of the University Hospital and School of Medicine. This step was provoked by a barrage of unjust criticism and unfair accusations which the governor launched against University Hospital authorities. In his letter Dr. Langston traced the origin of these attacks to several politically-minded, disgruntled employees. The next day Dean Long and Dr. Langston met with the regents to present their case, and the regents decided that two members of their board should confer with Governor Murray. The February 1 *Daily Oklahoman* stated that Governor Murray indicated that Dean Long was to stay. He also revealed that two persons, designated by him, had started to assemble information about the University Hospital immediately after the general election in 1930.

Later Dean Long received a letter dated March 20, from Dr. William H. Bailey, stating that he was trying to get the County Medical Society to pass a resolution supporting Dr. Long and Dr. Langston against "certain recent statements in the daily press, reporting testimony alleged to have been given before an investigation committee appointed by Governor Murray to check on the administration of the University Hospitals." Dean Long replied to Dr. Bailey's deduction that "dirty politics are being played," by saying that he was not being investigated personally.

Knowing that Dr. Langston would be unwilling to reconsider his resignation under the threatening circumstances, Dean Long again appeared before the regents on May 2, and asked that the former position of superintendent of the university hospitals be re-established. Two months later, on July 7, with President Bizzell and Dean Long present, the regents accepted the resignation of Dr. Wann Langston as administrative officer of the university hospitals and School of Medicine and forthwith appointed him professor of clinical medicine, as of September 1, 1931, on a half-time basis. Dr. Langston also succeeded Dr. Raymond Murdoch as director of the outpatient clinics and was appointed director of clinical clerkships. Hiram O. Moor was appointed executive assistant to the dean at this same meeting, and Dr. J. B. Smith, of

Durant, who formerly had been a legislative contact man for Governor Murray, became the new superintendent of the university hospitals on August 1, 1931. Three employees of the university hospitals were discharged for creating dissatisfaction and making threats against university officials.

Governor Murray, by dictatorial executive order, directed the authorities of the university to allow "any chiropractitioner" to practice in the University Hospital.[3]

The governor chose to interpret the intent of the 1917 legislative act providing for the construction of the University Hospital as a legal basis for chiropractors to attend patients there. That this action was part of a considered plan rather than the result of any sudden impulse can be deduced from a letter dated four months earlier, on March 16, 1931, and addressed to Governor Murray by Dr. N. P. Colwell, secretary of the Council on Medical Education and Hospitals:

"A rather alarming rumor has come to us that apparently measures are being contemplated which would take away from the teaching faculty of the University of Oklahoma control over the teaching material of the State University Hospital. We trust sincerely that this movement has not gone so far but that it can be corrected."

Dr. Colwell further stated that it was of utmost importance to the State of Oklahoma that the medical school should continue to control the teaching material in order to remain in the class of those schools whose standards meet requirements. "We would like to call your attention to the need of further financial support for your state medical school in order that it maintain its high standard . . . rather than in any way weakening the clinical teaching, . . ." he continued. "The University of Oklahoma School of Medicine has been making a valiant fight for improvements, particularly since your present dean was appointed, and it would indeed be unfortunate should that growth be in any way hindered at this time."

The governor's executive order, issued four months subsequent

[3] For a copy of this executive order, dated July 27, 1931, see Appendix III.

248

to Dr. Colwell's dictum, can be attributed solely to the machinations of a marplot. Indeed, as far away as Oregon his executive order was extolled on September 13 by a chiropractor in an *Oregonian* advertisement, which disclosed that Dr. O. S. Witt of the Carver Chiropractic College in Oklahoma City was the one who was admitted to practice in the University Hospital by executive order. The advertisement also quoted the governor as saying that Dr. Long's resignation would be "a damned good thing" and that he had plans in readiness to replace the entire faculty.

In answer to a September 14, 1931, inquiry from Dr. C. J. McCusker of the State Board of Medical Examiners in Oregon, Dr. L. J. Moorman reported that the particular patient involved died after a few days, which coincided with the prognosis made earlier by clinical faculty members of the School of Medicine.

Dean Long called a meeting of the faculty of the School of Medicine on July 27, and read Governor Murray's executive order, which had been issued the same day. Dr. Horace Reed was nominated as chairman by those present and was authorized to appoint a committee to draft a clear statement of precisely what the calculable risks of implementing the governor's executive order entailed. On August 1, the Council of the Oklahoma State Medical Association met and appointed a committee for the purpose of urging the regents of the university to hold an emergency session, but President Bizzell advised the committee that the regents felt that the matter should be postponed while an effort was made to "smooth things over."[4]

No doubt one reason for the regents' hesitancy was the fact that President Bizzell had earlier, on March 16, 1931, requested an attorney general's opinion on Section 6 of House Bill 366,[5] as it applied to the medical cults. He received the opinion on March 20 "that practitioners of osteopathy or chiropractic, duly licensed and regulated in accordance with the laws of this state, are entitled to the use of the State University Hospital as a place for treatment of

---

[4] *Journal of the Oklahoma State Medical Association*, Vol. XXIV (September, 1931), 311.

[5] *Session Laws*, 1917, Chapter 170, 299.

patients." Note that this opinion was dated exactly four days after Dr. Colwell's letter to Governor Murray warning of the consequences of such an eventuality to the teaching hospitals of the University of Oklahoma.

One can merely speculate as to what President Bizzell was thinking about between March 20, when he received the attorney general's opinion, and July 27, when the governor's executive order zeroed in on the university hospitals. In an August 1 letter to Dean Long, President Bizzell said that he had carefully reviewed the attorney general's opinion and that he was "afraid that the larger purposes of the hospital cannot escape the specific provision in Section 6, which states definitely that 'no rule or regulation shall prohibit the use of the hospital to any licensed physicians or surgeons not connected with the medical college'. . . . I realize that you made every possible effort to correct this serious situation, and I am inexpressibly sorry that the Governor could not see fit to approve the bill that was designed to correct this defect. . . . In view of this situation, I think we must look to some other temporary solution of the problem that will safeguard the integrity of our Medical School until we can secure the passage of a law that will forever settle this vexatious problem." Whatever the president thought it is apparent that he did not fully realize the urgency of a situation which could not be alleviated by any temporary solution.

From August 1 to August 4, letters and telegrams arrived for Dean Long and President Bizzell from Dr. Franklin H. Martin, director general, and Dr. Malcolm T. MacEachern, director of hospital activities, of the American College of Surgeons and from Dr. Olin West, secretary of the American Medical Association, notifying them that attendance on patients by chiropractors was in violation of the standards of class A medical school hospitals. They also stated that the attendance of chiropractors would make it necessary for the Council on Medical Education and Hospitals to remove the University of Oklahoma hospitals from the approved list and that disqualification of the School of Medicine would be the inevitable result.

According to Dean Long, the chiropractor was still coming to the hospital, and the School of Medicine would make no compromises. The governor agreed to leave the entire matter to the regents of the university, as the law required, but President Bizzell advised again, on August 6, that he was unable to get the regents to convene.

On August 7, Dean Long presided at a faculty meeting of the School of Medicine for the last time. He gave a brief résumé of the recent events and spoke of the acute situation in which the School of Medicine had been placed. Dean Long then called for the report of Dr. Horace Reed's committee. Dr. Reed said that the committee had met with Dean Long in the morning and that later in the day he had conferred with President Bizzell and Dean Long. The president told him that there were certain matters which would prove embarrassing to the regents if they should take action at this time, and he proposed to call on the School of Medicine's accrediting authorities in Chicago.

The following resolution was then read by Dr. Reed and adopted unanimously by the faculty.

"BE IT RESOLVED by the Faculty in session that we absolutely concur in the stand taken by Dr. Long, Dean of the School of Medicine—that the care of patients in the University and Crippled Children's Hospitals be limited entirely to the regular medical profession, since these hospitals were conceived and built as a laboratory for the teaching of clinical medicine in the University of Oklahoma School of Medicine.

"BE IT FURTHER RESOLVED that, in the interest of the medical students who are seriously disturbed and involved by the situation, the President and the Board of Regents be urged to take the earliest possible action toward solving the problem necessary to preserve our rating as an A Class medical school with approved hospitals for the training of interns.

SIGNED: FACULTY COMMITTEE:
Dr. Horace Reed, Chairman
Dr. E. S. Ferguson
Dr. G. A. LaMotte"

251

Dean Long again took the chair and declared that the governor of the state had made it impossible for him to perform his functions as dean and that he would forward his resignation to the president of the university in the morning as a protest against such interference with the school. "I resent the actions of the Governor and the Board of Regents, who should take steps to protect us." In his letter of resignation Dean Long explained:

"Because of the intolerable situation due to the action of the Governor in issuing an executive order to admit a member of one of the cults to University Hospital to treat a patient in our teaching service, and to the obvious unwillingness of the Board of Regents to take any early steps to correct the situation, notwithstanding our earnest and urgent requests, and the urgent and earnest requests of the State Medical Association, through you, I am placed in a position where it is impossible for me to properly perform the functions of the dean of the School of Medicine, an important part of this function being the supervision of work in the hospitals. . . .

"After carefully, deliberately and sadly thinking over the whole matter, I regret to have to advise you that, under the circumstances, it will be impossible for me to continue my duties. I, therefore, hand you my resignation from the position of Dean of the School of Medicine and from the position of Professor of Surgery and Head of the Department of Surgery, effective immediately."

After Dean Long's resignation was received on August 8, it was promptly announced that there would be a meeting of the regents on August 12. Meanwhile, President Bizzell made a hurried visit to representatives of the Council on Medical Education and Hospitals, the Association of American Medical Colleges, and the American College of Surgeons in Chicago. He was informed by all of them that the School of Medicine must be kept free of political influences to merit its A rating.

The Oklahoma State Medical Association had a weapon, too. At the request of its council, ex-justice of the supreme court, Thomas H. Owen, prepared a brief stating that under the law the cults could not be admitted to the University Hospital. As the basis for his opinion he cited a phrase in an appropriation act, "for equipment and supplies purchased for the Medical School and *hospital operated and maintained as a department of said State University.*"[6] He also called attention to House Bill No. 366, "an act providing $200,000 for construction of a hospital and buildings *for the Medical Department of the University of Oklahoma.*"[7]

The alumni were alerted to the gravity of the situation at the medical center by a letter written by Dr. Leonard C. Williams in August, 1931, on behalf of the board of directors of the alumni association of the School of Medicine. Dr. Williams explained that the hospital, as well as the School of Medicine, would lose its rating and that the dean and the entire faculty of the Medical School were prepared to resign their official positions in order to save the reputation of the medical profession. Alumni were requested to write to Governor Murray or to George L. Bowman, chairman of the board of regents of the university, expressing their opinions.

Representatives of several groups concerned about the plight of the University of Oklahoma School of Medicine appeared before the board of regents at the medical school on August 12, with President Bizzell in attendance. An Oklahoma State Medical Association committee (Drs. McClean Rogers, of Clinton; J. C. Fulton, of Atoka; and H. C. Webber, of Bartlesville) appeared and stated that the Oklahoma Medical Association was fighting for a principle in condemning the executive order.

Another committee, speaking for the faculty of the School of Medicine (Drs. E. S. Ferguson, George A. LaMotte, Horace Reed, and J. B. Smith) was also heard. These representatives stressed the importance of immediate action to safeguard the future status of the medical school.

6 *Extraordinary Session Laws*, 1916, Senate Bill No. 30, Chapter 12, 13.

7 According to a report prepared by Dean Lewis J. Moorman in 1935, there was a subsequent ruling by the attorney general confirming this interpretation that chiropractors could not be admitted to practice in the University Hospital without the approval of the regents. The validity of this opinion was afterward affirmed by the state supreme court.

A third committee, representing the osteopaths, appeared and submitted a statement claiming gross unfairness in their exclusion from hospitals.

Finally a committee consisting of Dr. H. K. Speed, of Sayre, whose son was a student in the School of Medicine, and two medical students, W. A. Minsch and T. L. Wainright, appeared on behalf of the student body of the medical school to express their deep concern over the prevailing difficulties. Chairman Bowman of the regents assured them that everything possible would be done to safeguard the School of Medicine.

The following resolution, drafted by Raymond A. Tolbert of Oklahoma City, and Joe C. Looney of Wewoka, was presented and approved by a five to two vote of the regents.

"*Whereas*, the University Hospital, was created primarily for the purpose of giving the required training and instruction to the medical students in the School of Medicine of the University of Oklahoma, and was placed under the jurisdiction and control of the Board of Regents of the University of Oklahoma as part of the University of Oklahoma, and,

"*Whereas*, it is necessary to restrict the use of said hospital to the doctors of medicine for practice therein in order to maintain the standing of said medical school, and,

"*Whereas*, it was the intent of the Legislature of Oklahoma in creating the University Hospital, to restrict the same to the use of doctors of medicine for practice therein;

"*Now Be It Resolved*, that the privileges of the University Hospital shall at all times be extended to any doctor of medicine, now or hereafter licensed or authorized to practice medicine by Chapter 59, Session Laws of Oklahoma, 1923.

"*Be It Further Resolved* that any patient or inmate in the University Hospital shall have the right at any time to select and receive treatment from any doctor of medicine as above defined."

A substitute resolution proffered by regents Claude C. Hatchett of Durant and Malcolm E. Rosser, Jr. of Muskogee, which would have permitted osteopaths and chiropractors in the University Hospital, failed by a vote of five to two. It is most interesting to note that only two of the five persons appointed to the board of regents by Governor Murray supported his executive order regarding the University Hospital.

President Bizzell presented the resignations of Dean Long and his two sons, Dr. LeRoy Downing Long and Dr. Wendell McLean Long, to the board. The resignations were accepted. The president then recommended that Dr. Lewis J. Moorman, an estimable member of the medical profession, be appointed the new dean, effective September 1, 1931, "until a full time Dean is secured."[8] The regents approved this recommendation.

Dean Long felt very strongly that he should not violate the pledge he had made when he was appointed dean of the University of Oklahoma School of Medicine in 1915. He had pledged that, as long as he was dean of the school, he would uphold the regulations and ideals of the Council on Medical Education and that, if any circumstances should arise that would make that course of action impossible, he would retire. As someone has said, "To know an ethical principle was for Dr. Long to make it a part of his life." Certainly one of the most important events in the history of the University of Oklahoma School of Medicine was the remarkable record of Dean Long's administration over a period of sixteen years. During this span the school gained financial support, built its first worthwhile physical facilities, saw the restoration of its class A rating, and became the nucleus for a future, expanded medical center.

Harlow's Weekly commented on these events in the issue of August 15, 1931. "At the time of the controversy between the Governor and members of the medical profession . . . over the chiropractic order, the Governor announced that a solution of the problem would be checked to the Board of Regents of the University, which has supervision over the hospital. Meeting in Oklahoma City last Wednesday, the Regents ruled against the

8 This was not an idle phrase, since in 1935, Dr. Leonard C. Williams, president of the Medical Alumni Association, testified to a senate committee that the association recommended the appointment of a full-time dean. Dr. Moorman's successor was appointed on that basis.

order admitting chiropractors, and held the institution was created and organized mainly as a strictly medical and surgical institution, and that, because of the difference in methods of treatment, members of the two professions could not well be accommodated in one institution. Following the action of the Regents, Governor Murray expressed the belief that the construction of a State Hospital, to which all representatives of all practices and theories of healing should be admitted, probably would ultimately be the solution of the controversy."

The *Journal of the Oklahoma State Medical Association* concluded that: "President Bizzell and the members of the Board of Regents were anxious to do everything legally possible in the interest of the School of Medicine, but . . . they were unable to understand the necessity of prompt action. . . . It seems impossible that the action of the Governor, or his interpretation of the law, has not done the University incalculable harm. . . . The entire performance has been one of the most unfortunate things that could occur to injure the medical school."[9]

What kind of man was Governor William H. Murray? He ruled by executive order in disregard of the legislature and the courts, and his first year of office was characterized as "a period of unbridled patronage, broken campaign promises and freak ideas."[10]

It might be sufficient to say that Governor Murray's interference in the School of Medicine was merely a phenomenon of demagogic politics, designed to arouse prejudices by sensational charges, specious arguments, and so on, and to gain political influence. Yet this does not quite explain the governor's Machiavellian harassment of institutions of higher learning. R. L. Luther, who included William H. Murray in his book *American Demagogues*, says that it is a demagogue's nature to fear college faculties and to regard professors as potential conspirators.[11] This gives one an inkling of why Governor Murray may have distrusted educated people. Luther calls these men egotistic professional "men of the people,"

9 *Journal of the Oklahoma State Medical Association*, Vol. XXIV (1931), 345.
10 *Oklahoma City Times*, January 12, 1932.
11 *American Demagogues, Twentieth Century* (Boston, Beacon Press, 1954).

of whom there were several in America during the first half of the twentieth century, all elected officials in various states.

"Alfalfa Bill" (also "Cocklebur Bill" and "Bolivia Bill") Murray was a talented exhibitionist who realized that an appreciable segment of the public preferred entertainment, display, and fanfare to solid information. He knew that the votes of those who delighted in showmanship would assist in his rise to power. For these people he was the "Sage of Tishomingo"; for those working in the medical center he was the "Enemy of the School of Medicine." It is true that he did not openly insist on removing Dean Long, whom he tormented, leaving the final decision concerning his executive order to the board of regents; but neither did Governor Murray openly relinquish his stand. Harassment was part of his political craftiness. As one senator commented at the time, "The most powerful dictatorial person in the State organization is your Governor. . . . He has a powerful political machine that will be hard to break. . . . I don't believe the Governor is going to pass anything that is detrimental to the doctors but he has the most retaliative reasoning of any man. You can't reason with him and you have got to catch him in the right mood. . . . There are in the Senate twenty-two rubber stamp men."[12]

It must be admitted that these "twenty-two rubber stamp men" helped pass several commendatory pieces of legislation during Murray's term of office, creation of the tax commission, the county excise board, the corporate income tax, and the furnishing of textbooks for school children.

1931 was a stormy year. It is hard to picture two more opposite personalities than Dean LeRoy Long, the protagonist, and Governor William H. Murray, the antagonist, moving in Oklahoma's limelight. Yet the history of any period is inseparable from politics, political men, and political forces, and we must never forget that another governor, Robert Williams, helped mightily to lay the first cornerstone of the Medical Center which Dean Long served so honorably. Development of the Southwest would move on very rapidly in the next quarter century, telescoping many advances into

[12] *Journal of the Oklahoma State Medical Association*, Vol. XXVI (1933), 214.

its recent history, while "Alfalfa Bill" Murray would be relegated to the position of a legendary character, together with the outlaws in the hills and the political escapades on an untamed frontier. The University of Oklahoma School of Medicine would continue to develop into a monument to those men and women of vision, dedication, and faith, who worked to build a first-class educational institution for the medical profession and its allied services.

We can now turn to the less traumatic events of the year. After Dr. Lewis J. Moorman became the succeeding dean of the School of Medicine on September 1, 1931, the political pressure by the governor lessened somewhat. Dr. Moorman was born near Leitch-field, Kentucky, in 1875. He graduated from Georgetown College in Kentucky in 1898 and received his M.D. degree from the University of Louisville in 1901, the same year in which he began his practice of medicine in Jet, Oklahoma. Subsequently, he undertook postgraduate study at New York Polyclinic Hospital, the University of Virginia, and the University of Vienna.

Dr. Moorman founded the College Sanatorium (later called the Farm Sanatorium) in Oklahoma City. He was appointed professor of physical diagnosis at the University of Oklahoma in 1910, and professor of clinical medicine in 1925. Dr. Moorman became a nationally known specialist on tuberculosis and chest diseases. He served as president of the Southern Medical Association, the American Trudeau Society, the National Tuberculosis Association, the Oklahoma State Medical Association, and the Oklahoma City Academy of Medicine. He was the author of four books of a historical nature.

By an act of the legislature the dean of the School of Medicine was made a member of a new appeal board created to consider appeals from licensure denial by the Oklahoma State Board of Medical Examiners.

At the July 7, 1931 meeting of the Board of Regents of the University of Oklahoma, President Bizzell reported that the State Board of Affairs had surrendered the former lease of a dairy farm west of Oklahoma City, which was operated for the University

Hospital, and had leased approximately one thousand acres seventeen miles northeast of the city for the same purpose.

Dean Moorman met with the faculty on September 18, when President Bizzell reported briefly on his visit with committees of the various accrediting agencies in Chicago. A discussion, as to whether part-time instructors in the medical school should be permitted to enroll in medical courses for credit, resulted in the opinion that the determination of this question should be left to the discretion of the dean and the heads of departments. A recommendation passed that students from junior colleges who intended to make application for entrance to the School of Medicine should be required to take an additional year in a recognized senior college before making application for admission to the medical school.

In a letter of September 21, Dean Moorman informed Harry C. Smith, business manager of the University Hospital, "I have arranged with the city manager to permit the City Health Department to occupy the first and second floors of the building at Third and Stiles Streets, since we hold the building on a 99 year lease."[13]

During the 1930–31 fiscal year, 6,509 patients were admitted to the University Hospital and 8,990 outpatients received 42,886 treatments. There were 2,907 admissions to the Hospital for Crippled Children. At this time the main University Hospital had approximately 225 beds, and the Crippled Children's Hospital 200 beds.[14] St. Anthony Hospital was listed in the 1931–32 university catalog as an affiliate of the School of Medicine. Kitty Shanklin was the director of social work in 1931, when that department began to function at the Hospital for Crippled Children.

The regents approved admission without charge for faculty members of the School of Medicine and professional members of

13 It was later in 1931 that P. B. Bostic was placed in charge of nonmedical personnel and business affairs by a resolution of the regents which made him directly responsible to them, thus eliminating the dean of the School of Medicine from this chain of authority. This arrangement was unwise and divisive, and it introduced a very disturbing element into Dr. Moorman's administration.

14 The Council on Medical Education and Hospitals reported a total of 447 beds in 1931.

the University Hospital organization as patients at the University Hospital. Free hospital care for nonprofessional employees was limited to two weeks.

According to the university catalog, the support for the university in 1931–32 was $1,581,638 and that for the medical campus was $581,744. The monies were distributed as follows: School of Medicine, $94,035; University Hospital, $308,521; and Hospital for Crippled Children, $179,187. The regents of the university subsequently reduced these amounts somewhat, according to the 1932–33 catalog.[15] It was estimated that the free medical and surgical services performed by the volunteer staff of physicians that year amounted to approximately $750,000.

Dr. N. P. Colwell resigned as secretary of the Council on Medical Education and Hospitals in 1931. The inspection of the University of Oklahoma School of Medicine was made in the fall for the council by Dr. E. A. Rygh. The report on the inspection, dated December 7, specified that the postgraduate program should be encouraged and that it should be directed by the medical school authorities rather than by the extension division of the university. The administration of the University Hospital was described as "not all that might be desired."

During the academic year 1931–32 there were 147 members of the faculty of the School of Medicine. Those newly appointed included Harry Wilkins, M.D., associate professor of surgery; Charles Nelson Berry, M.D., assistant professor of surgery; Howell Wesley Butler, M.D., assistant professor of histology, organology, and embryology; Joseph Benjamin Goldsmith, Ph.D., assistant professor of histology and embryology; Karl James Haig, M.D., assistant professor of anatomy; Mary Virginia Sawyer Sheppard, B.A., assistant professor of bacteriology; William Lawrence Bonham, M.D., instructor in otorhinolaryngology; John Flack Burton, M.D., instructor in surgery; Louis Harry Charney, M.D., instructor in medicine; Lee Kenneth Emenhiser, M.D., instructor in anatomy;

---

15 There was a reduction of approximately $45,000 from the medical campus budget, which had previously been decreased by $107,000 by the legislature from their 1929–30 appropriation.

Edmund Gordon Ferguson, M.D., instructor in ophthalmology; Floyd Gray, M.D., instructor in obstetrics; Wilma Jeanne Green, B.A., instructor in pathology; Hugh Clifford Jones, M.D., instructor in gynecology; James Floyd Moorman, M.D., instructor in medicine; Patrick Sarsfield Nagle, M.D., instructor in surgery; Tony Willard Pratt, M.S., instructor in physiology; James Robert Reed, M.D., instructor in anatomy; John Harrison Robinson, M.D., instructor in obstetrics; Fenton Almer Sanger, M.D., instructor in surgery; and Margaret Waddell, G.N., instructor in operating room technique. Ruth Thompson Hughes was appointed librarian for the School of Medicine in 1931, to succeed Mrs. Grace Swain Cassidy, who retired.

In the 1931–32 bulletin for the School of Medicine is a description of the series of elective courses. Each student was required to select 160 clock hours of electives during the last three years of study, distributed as follows: second year, 16 hours; third year, 48 hours, and fourth year, 96 hours. Honor students were permitted to substitute 112 hours of their research work for an equal amount of elective courses. The committee in general charge of the electives consisted of Professors J. T. Martin, R. M. Howard, and M. R. Everett. The dean of the School of Medicine appointed three additional committees to advise students of the last three years on elective selection. A total of 412 clock hours of elective courses was offered.

Forty-three medical students graduated with M.D. degrees in 1931. Among them were Jack Paul Birge, Ned Burleson, Phil J. Devanney, Lee Kenneth Emenhiser, James William Finch, Onis George Hazel,[16] Jess Duval Hermann, Wilbur Floyd Keller, John Frederick Kuhn, Jr., Cecil Willard Lemon, A. C. Little, Welborn W. Sanger, and C. Donovan Tool. In the 1931–32 academic year there were 238 students in the School of Medicine and 141 in the School of Nursing. Twenty-three graduates of the School of Nursing received the degree of graduate nurse.

It is interesting to note at this point that during the first thirty-two

16 Onis Hazel was one of the charter members of the Toga, a senior honor society organized in 1922 on the Norman campus for students in professional schools.

years of the existence of the School of Medicine 509 M.D. degrees were granted, and in the first nineteen-year period of the School of Nursing, 238 graduate nurses received certificates.

T. M. Beaird, from the university extension division, reported that twenty-one counties had been reached through the postgraduate medical teaching program during the year and that 917 physicians and surgeons had attended courses. A newly introduced film program was considered very successful, too.[17]

The Council of the Oklahoma State Medical Association appointed Dr. L. S. Willour and Dr. F. H. McGregor to co-operate with the committee on postgraduate medical instruction of the State University. It also provided $350 to help underwrite visits by four outstanding medical authorities to appear in six of the largest cities of the state for one-day clinics. Dr. C. B. Francisco of Kansas City, Missouri, was engaged to conduct a postgraduate course on traumatic and orthopedic surgery with accompanying fracture clinics.

[17] For other complimentary statements see the *Journal of the Oklahoma State Medical Association*, Vol. XXIV (1931), 55, 175, 200, 204, 410.

XIV. Epilogue

DR. LEROY LONG continued to be active in his private surgical practice and in the profession generally, from 1931 until his death on October 27, 1940. He was president of the Oklahoma City Academy of Medicine in 1932, of the Oklahoma Academy of Science, and of the Oklahoma State Medical Association in 1934–35. In 1936 he was inducted into the Oklahoma Hall of Fame.

Dr. Long was survived by two sons in the medical profession, Dr. LeRoy Downing Long, clinical professor of surgery at the School of Medicine, who died in 1970, and Dr. Wendell McLean Long, an instructor in gynecology, who resigned in 1931 and died in 1946. Three of Dean Long's grandchildren also became physicians, Dr. LeRoy Long III, instructor in surgery at the Medical Center, Dr. Lyda Long, and Dr. Wendell Long II.

An oil portrait of Dean LeRoy Long, which hangs in the library of the School of Medicine, was presented by alumni and friends of the dean in early October, 1931. There is a letter in the dean's files, dated October 10, 1931, from Dean Moorman to Dr. Long, acknowledging the receipt of a "letter of appreciation in connection with the portrait, which was presented to the School of Medicine at the last Clinical Society meeting, and to say that it is being held for presentation at the next Faculty meeting."

The following are abstracts from some of the many eulogies that were spoken and written after the passing of Dr. LeRoy Long.

"He rendered great beneficial and distinguished service to the state. It was whilst he was Dean of the Medical School that the site,

263

on which the medical department is located, was set aside for such purpose, and all of the buildings and the greater part of the equipment therein were constructed and acquired. . . . The medical school is a monument to his leadership."[1]

"Were I a preacher looking for a text upon which to base a sermon on the subject of the ideal physician, I would feel that I have in the life and works of Dr. LeRoy Long, the fullness of a text personified. . . . His wise counsel has often been sought and accepted by organized medicine in this state, and he invariably has stood for the things that were right, irrespective of any extraneous influence. His judicious mind and his high ethical standards were always the basis for sound conclusions. . . . No doubt the master accomplishment of his career was the development of our medical school. . . . He was a wonderful teacher, as can be attested by many of us who sat at his feet . . . he taught all with whom he came in contact by precept and example, a high standard of ethics, and a righteous mode of living."[2]

"[Dr. Long] served his profession with unquestionable skill, always conditioned by unfailing loyalty and wisdom. . . . His character was above reproach. . . ." This obituary also described his "striking appearance, his dignified demeanor, his ready speech, his sense of propriety, and his professional attainments. . . ." It continued, "In the death of Dr. Long the medical profession has lost a great champion of industry, courtesy, honor and integrity. . . . these sterling attributes of character have a spiritual value which should become an abiding influence on the lives of those who are left behind."[3]

"A sincere and consecrated man . . . a guide and a pillar of strength is gone from the councils of organized medicine. . . . his gentle manner and great human kindliness combined with an air

1 Judge Robert L. Williams, former governor of Oklahoma and president of the Oklahoma Historical Society, in a letter, November 18, 1940.

2 Dr. L. S. Willour, in a eulogy at the 1940 annual banquet of the Oklahoma County Medical Association.

3 "Obituary," *Journal of the Oklahoma State Medical Association*, Vol. XXXIII (December, 1940), 34.

of mastery, inspired confidence and hope in the patient. Dr. Long did not seek prominence or position. . . . It would have been difficult to have found a man better qualified [to become Dean of the School of Medicine]. . . . It was a situation where, amid fast moving events, progress had to be made. . . . Conservatism and a firm grip were the qualities necessary at the helm. These qualities Dr. Long possessed to a remarkable degree. . . . He had an unquestioning faith in those he trusted . . . came to his conclusions after thought and deliberation. . . . yet he was capable of quick decisions in cases of emergency. . . . Dr. Long was a great reader. . . . his presence created an atmosphere more eloquent than a sermon. . . . A man of highest ethical standards and one who lived his convictions, an inspiring teacher, an efficient administrator, a learned counselor . . . a loyal friend, a man who with modesty and humility built for himself a high place in the medical world. . . ."[4]

"The services rendered to this school and to the State of Oklahoma by this outstanding man can not be too highly valued; that during sixteen years as Dean of the University of Oklahoma School of Medicine this institution was raised from a mediocre standing to one of the best medical schools in the United States; that his professional and executive ability were the propelling forces in this advancement; that during his tenure of office he saw the building of the present University and Crippled Children's Hospitals; and that it is our opinion that those institutions will long stand as a monument of the accomplishments of our beloved Dr. LeRoy Long.

"We feel that in his passing we have lost a true friend, a benefactor of mankind, a loyal and forceful medical administrator, a surgeon of the greatest skill, a man of courage imbued with the conviction that justice and honesty are the highest attributes of mankind; that he will long live in our memory and feel that his record will be an inspiration and serve as a model for those who follow him in the practice of medicine; that his name will be

4 Dr. L. A. Turley, "LeRoy Long, Doctor and Educator," *Sooner Magazine*, Vol. XIII, No. 4 (1940), 18.

perpetuated in this institution as a guide for present and future members, and that by his life and character the community has benefited to the highest degree. . . ."[5]

An annual LeRoy Long Lectureship was instituted at the school in 1941 by the Alpha Lambda Chapter of the Phi Beta Pi medical fraternity, with Dr. Ernest Sachs, professor of clinical neurosurgery in Washington University School of Medicine, as the first lecturer.

On May 18, 1941, a bronze memorial tablet, donated by the Oklahoma State Medical Association, was dedicated in the auditorium of the School of Medicine Building to the memory of Dean Long. It was placed in the south lobby of the building. The wording on the memorial tablet is particularly appropriate to a distinguished dean, "Kind and Understanding Doctor—Builder of the Medical School—Courageous Leader of Ethical and Scientific Medicine."

It is the historian's unique privilege to give balanced thought and proper interpretation to the events he portrays. He can, for example, trace the evolutionary progress and appraise the significance of changes in medical education over a period of time better than the casual observer. Many of those interested in suggesting innovations and changes in medical education could benefit by devoting some of their attention to the past history of the subject, thus saving themselves from frustrating experiments. There indeed is a common tendency for young energetic teachers to regard their own thoughts as original ones, whereas they frequently prove to be ventures that have already been tried and proven defective in one respect or another. There are fads in medical education as in any other line of human endeavor. When such fads are widely accepted they tend to create uniformity in schools of medicine.

Certainly it was not by chance that those who envisioned a University of Oklahoma Medical Center were able to develop a creditable institution at the turn of the century. Any School of Medicine at Norman could scarcely have survived prior to 1900, because even the four-year bachelor's program in the arts and

[5] Resolution from the faculty of the School of Medicine, January 28, 1941.

sciences was not effective until 1898, when bachelor's degrees were granted to the two first graduates.

The early youthful deans of the School of Medicine organized an entirely acceptable curriculum for the two-year school. By 1906 the school was accorded membership in the Association of American Medical Colleges. Three years later the university, through its Graduate College, was able to offer graduate study in the basic medical sciences. Considering the very low national status of medical education prior to 1910, these accomplishments represented remarkable progress for a fledgling medical school and its small parent university.

One resource that provided encouragement to the new medical school was the intelligent interest of physicians in Oklahoma City in developing a four-year School of Medicine. Several medical practitioners attempted unsuccessfully in 1903 to interest the University of Oklahoma in adding the last two clinical years to its medical school. Similar efforts continued from time to time, but it required seven more years and the publication of the *Flexner Report* to bring such a plan to fruition. The very great influence of the *Flexner Report* came at a most opportune time for the University of Oklahoma School of Medicine. It established a sound and approved basis for the merger of the Epworth College of Medicine (class C) into the newly expanded four-year school of the University of Oklahoma (class A).

The School of Medicine, which survived the rigors of territorial days and the disturbances generated during the terms of the first two pioneer governors of the state of Oklahoma, was soon faced with a new ten-year struggle to justify an A rating by overcoming its total lack of facilities for clinical training. There were many new and challenging responsibilities for the largely volunteer faculty, not the least of which was the necessity of providing the essential teaching hospital facilities.

Over the years the belief became widespread that the entire clinical faculty of the Epworth College of Medicine took part in the formation of the new school and that the entire University of

Oklahoma clinical faculty was composed of former Epworth staff members. Actually, only half of the Epworth faculty volunteered to join the University School of Medicine, but fortunately there were other capable physicians in Oklahoma City who wanted to assist in the instruction of young medical students.

The expansion of the School of Medicine to a four-year program in 1910 was a historic action by the State Regents of the University of Oklahoma, which they undertook without any immediate or promised financial aid or legislative assistance. Their wise and courageous decision deserves praise.

The year 1911 became a year of firsts. There was the first agitation to build a university hospital, stemming from the medical profession itself. There was also the first recorded meeting of the faculty of the School of Medicine and the faculty's action to start a School of Medicine library.

A new State Board of Education, replacing the State Board of Regents for the university, was authorized by the legislature at the request of Governor Cruce in 1911. It was subject to much criticism, and it inherited a very annoying situation at the School of Medicine. Nevertheless, the new board undertook to help the school in certain ways. Most of its actions were not divulged to the faculty, such as the employment of a capable consultant, Dr. Augustus G. Pohlman, to advise the board in regard to the organization and development of the four-year school. His recommendations proved to be very wholesome and timely, but they were adopted only in part and were put into effect at all too slow a pace.

In 1911 the first fifteen M.D. degrees were conferred by the University of Oklahoma. At that time it was customary to employ a registered nurse as hospital superintendent, and Miss Annette B. Cowles performed this duty. The University Hospital was housed in Oklahoma City in Rolater Hospital, which had been rented from Dr. Joseph B. Rolater in 1911. Dr. Robert Findlater Williams of Richmond, Virginia, became dean of the School of Medicine.

The next year, 1912, witnessed the appointment of a very effective president of the university, Dr. Stratton D. Brooks. Elected by the State Board of Education, President Brooks developed into a worthy friend and advocate of the medical school. The year also witnessed the occupation of the newly rented State University Hospital and its outpatient department. President Brooks established the principle of county reimbursement for the care of indigent patients at the University Hospital. The School for Nurses opened.

It was soon apparent that Dean Williams was not an experienced university administrator, since he managed to dishearten the volunteer portion of his faculty by eliminating and demoting worthy faculty members with insufficient cause. This action unfortunately overshadowed his better accomplishments. Moreover the School of Medicine was reclassified as a B school in 1912. Dean Williams resigned early in 1913. He was followed by two local physicians in succession, who were reputable practitioners but devoid of the qualities necessary for effective administration of the school.

In 1913, Dr. Francis B. Fite, of Muskogee, was appointed to the State Board of Education. He soon emerged as part of the hardworking triumvirate, consisting of Governor Williams, Dean Long, and Dr. Fite, which secured an appropriation for the new University Hospital in 1917. Earlier attempts by Dr. Fite to assist the School of Medicine were frustrated by administrative stagnation at the school. The Council on Medical Education recommended in 1914 that the university erect its own hospital building, with a warning that otherwise the rating of its School of Medicine could not be improved.

The five-year stalemate, from 1911 to 1915, ended when Governor Williams allocated funds to the School of Medicine in 1915 for equipment. The State Board of Education executed a lease on a second hospital, the Oklahoma City General Hospital, to provide quarters for the School of Medicine. In 1916 the governor arranged a deficiency allocation for the School of Medicine. He recommended an appropriation of $200,000 for the new hospital. The Tulsa County Medical Society helped considerably at this stage by boosting the governor's proposal.

Dean Long, having acquired sufficient backing from the medical profession and the active support of Governor Williams, took up the gauntlet in 1916 in a drive to erect a new University Hospital in Oklahoma City, an objective that was achieved a year later. By this time Dr. Long had developed a very effective political philosophy and considerable skill in public contacts. He appreciated the need for public support and for informing the public. It was crystal clear to him that the construction of the University Hospital was the very essential first step to the entire future of the University of Oklahoma School of Medicine and its Medical Center.

With the completion of the new hospital in 1919, the faculty and the medical profession were greatly encouraged, for this accomplishment made possible the later medical developments at the university.

This goal was achieved despite the activities essential to efforts of the First World War, in which the Medical School's participation was very creditable; General Hospital No. 56 was located at the School of Medicine, as was the postwar care of veterans.

The new University Hospital was very properly placed by law under the regents of the University of Oklahoma, which replaced the State Board of Education as the governing board of the university. The direct administration of the hospital became a duty of the dean of the School of Medicine. While this teaching hospital was constructed partly as a resource for medical care of indigent patients of the state, the law wisely authorized the inclusion of a certain number of private beds, a fact which was quite generally forgotten by members of the medical profession in later years.

In 1918, Paul Fesler became the first manager and superintendent of the University Hospital following the three previous nurse superintendents. With the new University Hospital came the beginning of residencies and of a program of dietetics. Former Governor Williams, in late 1919, was the first to state that the School of Medicine should include a Department of Dentistry. This department was not created until some years later, and then as a subdivision of the Department of Surgery of the School of Medicine. It was a half century later that a separate School of Dentistry was organized.

The second State Board of Regents of the university, created by the legislature in 1919, proved to be the first stable governing

270

board, well protected by law from political events. The three former governing boards, during the first twenty years of the School of Medicine, had succumbed to political conditions for one reason or another, but the board formed in 1919 is still the governing board of the university today.

Dr. Wann Langston became the medical superintendent of the University Hospital in 1920, the year of the restoration of the University of Oklahoma School of Medicine to a class A status in recognition of the major building improvements, the better equipment, and the expansion of the basic science program in the School of Medicine. The formal announcement of the class A status was made on March 11, 1920. In his accompanying letter, Dr. Colwell urged that a new School of Medicine building be constructed. The Committee on Medical Education of the Oklahoma State Medical Association made a similar recommendation. An article in the 1920 *Journal of the Oklahoma State Medical Association* recalled the earlier "strange anomaly of opposition from a few members of the medical profession inspired by selfishness or pique," and it expressed the hope that never again should the school lack funds and support.

In 1921 the legislature provided $75,000 to create space for a veterans ward at the University Hospital. Also, in the legislative field, a successful campaign was waged to defeat a proposal permitting osteopaths to practice in the University Hospital and in other state and city hospitals.

A Nurses Home was constructed at the University Hospital in 1921. There was a marked increase in the number of applicants for entrance into the School of Medicine during the next few years, as expected from the re-establishment of the class A status and the availability of the new teaching hospital.

Physicians of the state were even then complaining of a lack of reports from the University Hospital on patients which they had referred to it. This chronic problem was to be encountered a number of times in the succeeding years. The reason for this failure is easy to determine. It was the inevitable result of insufficient stenographic and clerical help at the hospital to meet the requests

271

routinely and regularly. Moreover, this annoying problem was related to another which has been a prevalent defect of the staffs of numerous hospitals in years gone by, namely the completion of hospital charts on time. Such routine paperwork has always been a distasteful chore to the busy clinician.

1922 was marked by an increased number of applicants to the School of Nursing, which had also become a class A school. The laboratories of the University Hospital were improved markedly, and a hospital board consisting of faculty members was instituted.

In 1923, Dean Long exhorted the ninth legislature to build a School of Medicine building in Oklahoma City and to move the basic science departments there from Norman. "We have no permanent home at Norman," said Dean Long. The legislature did pass the appropriation, but earmarked it for the Norman campus, due largely to pressure exerted by certain Norman businessmen. A more successful act passed by this legislature was its first authorization of the medical and surgical treatment of indigent children, sponsored by Hon. Allen M. Street, Hon. James C. Nance, and Paul Fesler, all of whom were Rotarians interested in the Society for Crippled Children. The passage of this act set the stage for the future construction of a Children's Hospital at the University of Oklahoma campus in Oklahoma City. In connection with these progressive events in 1923, it should be noted that Governor Walton's term was too short to pose any real hindrance to the plans of the School of Medicine. Governor Trapp, who succeeded him, was able to create and maintain an encouraging atmosphere at the Capitol.

While regular graduate courses in the basic science departments had been offered since 1909, the programs of clinical courses for physicians began only in 1925, after being somewhat overdue. Such postgraduate courses were started then, and the honors course in research for medical students was also launched at that time.

Certain events in regard to the University Hospital had been developing for some few years and came to the fore in 1926. One of these was a legislative policy to make separate appropriations for the University Hospital apart from the appropriations to the rest of the university, but these were funneled through the regents. There is no doubt that this policy reduced arguments and irritations between the faculty and administration at Norman and at the Medical Center. In later years the separate budget was extended to the entire Oklahoma City campus.

In 1926, Paul Fesler declared a real need for a private pavilion to be built by public contributions at the University Hospital, but nothing was done about it. A threatening financial difficulty made its appearance in 1926 through the refusal by certain counties, including the Oklahoma County Commissioners, to reimburse the University Hospital for the cost of care of the county's indigent patients. This led to much argument in the legislature for a number of years.

The American Hospital Association suggested in 1926 that the dean of the School of Medicine be relieved of the direct administration of the University Hospital, since the combined task was regarded as too great for one person to discharge. It is interesting to recall that during the year Dean Long reported to the medical faculty a belief of the public that graduates of the School of Medicine were unwilling to locate in rural districts. This problem remains today. It is evident that it represents no fault of the medical schools. The protest has become even more insistent as the years have passed, since it actually is a facet of the nation-wide urbanization trend. Many suggestions and experiments have been made by American medical schools in attempt to counteract this tendency, but without great success.

Some of the most important events in the early history of the School of Medicine occurred in 1928, when the new School of Medicine building was constructed in Oklahoma City as well as the new Crippled Children's Hospital, the second University Hospital. Also there were the very distressing and discouraging events in 1931 which led to the resignation of Dean Long and a setback in the development of the School of Medicine and the Medical Center.

The growth of the University of Oklahoma School of Medicine and its contribution to the state can be best illustrated by comparing certain figures for 1900 and 1931. In 1900 there were three faculty members in the School of Medicine and eight medical students; in 1931 there were 147 faculty members, 238 medical students, and 141 students in the School of Nursing. In 1900 no patients were being cared for by the School of Medicine, while in the fiscal year 1930–31, 6,509 patients at the University Hospital, 2,907 patients at the Crippled Children's Hospital, and 8,990 patients in the out-patient departments received medical and surgical treatment. The budgets for the School of Medicine, its allied hospitals, and the School of Nursing were $1,300 in 1900, and $668,250 in 1930.[6]

In 1900 the School of Medicine occupied one small wooden building at Norman, but through the thirty-two years of its development to 1931, it made use of twenty-five different buildings, ten constructed by the university, ten owned by affiliated hospitals, and five rented temporarily. Of these, six university-owned buildings remained in use in 1931, including the two large hospitals and the School of Medicine building which took care of all the major activities on the Oklahoma City campus.

By 1931 a total of 509 physicians had graduated from the School of Medicine, and 238 nurses from the School of Nursing.

By and large, the faculty members were serious in the performance of their teaching and research duties, and the clinical members, most of whom gave their time voluntarily, were genuinely interested in developing those characteristics in students which would mold them into helpful, reliable, and considerate physicians. The faculty as a whole was continuously underpaid, but nevertheless its members constituted the real strength of the School of Medicine. They were the many who served the public and the university well, without praise or fortune.

The students on their part, were eager young people who had selected medicine as a life's work. In the earlier years they were comparatively poorly prepared to undertake medical studies, especially the medical sciences. However, the gradual increase in prerequisites in the form of required college courses did much to

6 Under Governor Murray the 1931 budget was reduced temporarily by approximately $150,000.

mature the medical student to a stage where he could master his medical studies efficiently. Both faculty and students were intrinsically very loyal to the School of Medicine and to the profession. Problems of discipline were few and far between.[7]

Looking back over the thirty-two years, it is interesting to recall how many workers, how many students, and how many scholars there were who elevated the environment and tone of the School of Medicine. Yet, with all their support, in times of stress, only a few effective leaders emerged who were able and willing to make the requisite effort to rescue the school from an uncertain future.

Some of the difficulties surmounted in the institution's survival were problems common to many schools of medicine. For example, reappearing perennially in discussions by legislators was the myth that the American Medical Association limited the number of medical students in training in order to control the size of the profession. Actually, the only control which the American Medical Association exerted, through its Council on Medical Education, was to establish proper training for students of medicine.

Our School of Medicine had some serious problems peculiar to the University of Oklahoma, namely the loss of two fine university presidents and the forced resignation of two effective deans, because of political pressures, during a period of thirty-two years. The last casualty of this sort was during the term of Governor Murray, for subsequent governors and legislators developed a more educated attitude toward our institutions of higher learning. Of course the School of Medicine moved forward despite the impediments contributed by Governor Murray, and, since nothing succeeds as well as success, favorable opinion toward the school gradually developed both on the part of the public and its legislators.

While all the deans of the School of Medicine, during the period considered in this volume, were part-time administrators and part-

[7] The author has made no attempt to present a complete list of students and graduates of the Medical Center who received the M.D., M.S., Ph.D., or G.N. degrees and certificates. The University of Oklahoma Office of Student Affairs, the associate dean of the Graduate College, and the dean of the School of Nursing have the official lists of all students and graduates on file.

time practitioners of medicine, this arrangement finally became a real problem, as was the case in many medical schools. An impending switch to full-time deans became evident during the final years of the period. In 1935, General Robert Urie Patterson was appointed as the first full-time dean at the University of Oklahoma School of Medicine.

The basic medical sciences exerted an increasing emphasis and significance on medical education and medical practice during the ten years prior to 1932. A scholarly atmosphere, inspirational teachers, and students having a desire to search the unknown were most important factors in the development of a School of Medicine. Medical education's attention to the newer discoveries made in the medical sciences, and their applications to medicine, marked the greatest step forward for the profession.

In conclusion, it should be pointed out that even though 1931 ended on a note of pessimism, a much greater destiny was to be the fortune of the School of Medicine in the years ahead when it would rise to heights greater than ever attained before. In 1932 the University of Oklahoma School of Medicine was well on its way to becoming a great medical center. The torch of learning, lighted by those very few in 1900, was passed on to ever younger hands that would continuously reconstitute an institution that existed not for its day alone, but for the future, worthy of its place near the pinnacle of the teaching art.

APPENDIX I The Academic Departments and Heads
of the School of Medicine and the
School of Nursing, Prior to 1932

From 1900 to 1906 most of the courses in the School of Medicine were under the supervision of the biology department, the chemistry department, and the School of Pharmacy of the university. The last teaching by the biology department terminated in 1918. While most instruction by the School of Pharmacy ended by 1906, its final teaching was in 1926. The chemistry department ended its instruction in 1924.

The anatomy department was the department first designated in the School of Medicine by the Territorial Board of Regents in 1900, but it actually operated as a division of the biology department of the university until 1905. Three additional departments were instituted in 1906, namely forensic medicine, pathology, and bacteriology and physiology. A report of the board of regents to Governor Haskell in 1907 states that these three departments together with the anatomy department and the Department of Chemistry were organized in the medical school in 1906.

The Department of Anatomy. This department began in 1900 with Dr. Lawrence Northcote Upjohn as head from 1900 to 1904. The succeeding heads of this department were: Roy Philson Stoops, M.D., 1904–1908; Walter Leander Capshaw, M.D., 1908–15; Reuben Morgan Hargrove, M.D., 1916–19; Joseph Clark Stephenson, Ph.D., M.D., 1919–31; and Carmen Russell Salsbury, M.D., 1931–33. At the time of the 1907 report to Governor Haskell the Department of Anatomy included histology. However, for the most of the period from 1906 to 1920 the subject of histology was taught by the Department of Pathology. A new Department of Histology and Embryology was formed in 1920, with Dr. Joseph Mario Thuringer as its head.

The Department of Chemistry. Edwin C. DeBarr, Ph.D., was the

277

head of this department in the School of Medicine from its inception in 1906 until 1923. It was in 1924 that a new Department of Biochemistry and Pharmacology was created in the School of Medicine, with Mark Reuben Everett, Ph.D., as head of the department. The new department took over the teaching duties of the chemistry department of the university and of the School of Pharmacy. In 1935 this joint department was separated into the departments of biochemistry and pharmacology. At that time Dr. Everett remained with the Department of Biochemistry as its head until 1964.

The Department of Forensic Medicine. This department, which lasted only from 1906 to 1910, had as its head Charles Sharp Bobo, M.D. It was purely a temporary department designed to solve some problems of the day.

The Department of Pathology and Bacteriology. Founded in 1906, this department had Edward Marsh Williams, B.S., as its first head, from 1906 to 1908. He was succeeded by Louis Alvin Turley, M.A., in 1909. Professor Turley continued as head of the Department of Pathology until 1944. Bacteriology split off as a new Department of Bacteriology and Hygiene in 1912.

The Department of Physiology. This department was the last to be instituted in 1906, and it actually had no head until John Dice Maclaren, M.D., was appointed in 1908. Dr. Roy Philson Stoops had previously been an instructor in physiology in 1903 prior to the formation of the department itself. The subject of pharmacology was at that time incorporated into the Department of Physiology. The heads of the physiology department were: John Dice Maclaren, M.D., 1908–11; Albert Clifford Hirshfield, M.D., 1911–12, Leonard Blain Nice, Ph.D., 1913–27; and Edward Charles Mason, M.D., Ph.D., 1928–50.

The Department of Bacteriology. Begun as a joint department with pathology in 1906, the Department of Bacteriology was first headed by Edward Marsh Williams, from 1906 to 1908. He was followed by Louis Alvin Turley, 1909–11. In 1912, a new Department of Bacteriology and Hygiene was formed separate from pathology. Gayfree Ellison, M.D., was head of this Department of Bacteriology and Hygiene from 1912 to 1928, after which he remained with the university in Norman, since he was director of the student infirmary there. Hiram Dunlap Moor, M.S., became head of the department in 1929 and remained in that position until 1951.

278

The University of Oklahoma School of Medicine became a four-year school in 1910. The clinical teaching during the year 1910–11 was conducted without any official departmental organization. By 1912 the new clinical departments were the Department of Medicine, Archa Kelly West, M.D., head, and the Department of Surgery, William James Jolly, M.D., head. Appointed also were heads for the specialty subdivisions of the two departments.

The Department of Medicine. In 1912 the Department of Medicine included the following specialty subdivisions: children's diseases, William Merritt Taylor, M.D.; nervous and mental disorders, Antonio Debord Young, M.D.; clinical laboratories, Casriel J. Fishman, M.D.; and genitourinary, skin, and venereal diseases, Curtis Richard Day, M.D. There were only two heads of the Department of Medicine prior to 1932, namely, Dr. Archa Kelly West, M.D., 1912–26, and George Althouse LaMotte, M.D., 1926–44.

The Department of Surgery. This department also had subdivisions: orthopedics, Robert Lord Hull, M.D.; eye, ear, nose, and throat diseases, Edmund Sheppard Ferguson, M.D.; gynecology, Robert Mayburn Howard, M.D.; obstetrics, John Archer Hatchett, M.D.; and radiography, Everett Samuel Lain, M.D. The heads of the Department of Surgery were as follows: William James Jolly, M.D., 1912; John William Riley, M.D., 1913–15; LeRoy Long, M.D., 1915–31; and Robert Mayburn Howard, M.D., 1931–43.

During the next four years these two large departments began to be fragmented. We shall consider the other departments in alphabetical order.

The Department of Anesthesiology. This department was not organized until 1930, at which time John Alfred Moffett, M.D., became its head, from 1930 to 1938. John Mosby Alford, M.D., was the first to serve as an anesthetist in the University Hospital, from 1911 to 1913. Alford instituted the first course in anesthetics for medical students in 1912 in the Department of Surgery. This course was given annually until 1923. From 1924 to 1928 the course in anesthetics was moved to the jurisdiction of the Department of Medicine, but in 1929 it was no longer taught. Floyd Jackson Bolend, M.D., was the second hospital anesthetist, from 1913 to 1915. He was appointed instructor and assistant professor in children's diseases, from 1912 to 1915, and became assistant professor of medicine in 1916, associate professor of medicine in 1923, and head of the hospital Department of Anesthesia

279

until 1930, at which time the School of Medicine's Department of Anesthesiology was formed. In the period 1935–37, both Dr. Moffett and Dr. Bolend were in the department. Only Dr. Moffett remained in 1938, Dr. Floyd Bolend having retired in 1937. Dr. Bolend was appointed emeritus head of the Department of Anesthesia in 1935.

The Department of Dermatology. In 1911–12, skin diseases were taught together with genitourinary and venereal diseases by Curtis Richard Day, M.D., as a subsection of medicine, while Everett Samuel Lain, M.D., was head of the subdivision of radiography at the same time. From 1913 to 1915 there was a similar grouping of skin diseases with venereal and genitourinary diseases under John William Riley, M.D., head of the department. However, in 1916, dermatology was separated from the other two subjects. It was taught in the Department of Dermatology, Electrotherapy, and Radiography by Dr. Everett S. Lain, who remained head of the department until 1942. In 1921 the department name changed from dermatology, electrotherapy, and radiography to dermatology, electrotherapy, and radiology. There was one further change in the name in 1935, to the Department of Dermatology, Radiology, and Roentgenology, and later that year when a separate Department of Radiology was formed, it became the Department of Dermatology.

The Department of Gynecology. Robert Mayburn Howard, M.D., was the head of this subsection of the Department of Surgery in 1912. Then in 1913–15 the Department of Obstetrics-Gynecology, with John Archer Hatchett, M.D., as head, was formed. The year 1916 showed a further change in the name of the department to gynecology, with John Smith Hartford, M.D., as the head. Dr. Hartford retained this position until 1924, at which time John Frederick Kuhn, M.D., became the head of the department until 1939.

The Department of Obstetrics. John Archer Hatchett, M.D., was head of this department from 1912 until 1933. In 1911–12 it was a subdivision of the Department of Surgery. It was part of the joint Department of Obstetrics-Gynecology in 1913–15. It returned to its separate department status in 1916 and then remained so.

The Department of Ophthalmology. The specialties, Eye, Ear, Nose, and Throat Diseases, subdivisions of the Department of Surgery 1912–15, became a joint department in 1913 with Edmund Sheppard Ferguson, M.D., as head. In 1916 two separate departments were formed, with Dr. Ferguson as head of the Department of Ophthalmology and

Lauren Haynes Buxton, M.D., as head of Ear, Nose, and Throat Diseases. In 1922 the two separate departments again became a joint department, with Dr. Ferguson as the head, 1922–24. The separate Department of Ophthalmology was then re-established, with Dr. Ferguson as the head, 1924–39.

The Department of Orthopedic Surgery. Orthopedic surgery did not become a department until 1936. However, until 1932 there were eight faculty members with titles related to orthopedic surgery in the department.

The Department of Otorhinolaryngology. From 1912 to 1915 otorhinolaryngology was a joint department with ophthalmology, with Dr. Edmund S. Ferguson as head. From 1916 until 1921 otorhinolaryngology was a separate department with Lauren Haynes Buxton, M.D., as its head. After Dr. Buxton's death in 1922, the joint department was re-established with Dr. Ferguson again as head. The final separation into a separate otorhinolaryngology department took place in 1924. H. Coulter Todd, M.D., was the head of this separate department until 1936.

The Department of Pediatrics. This department was established in 1930, with William M. Taylor, M.D., as the head until 1938. Before the separate department was formed, there were seven faculty members in the Department of Medicine who carried titles related to the subject of pediatrics, including Dr. Taylor himself.

The Department of Pharmacology. Prior to 1924 pharmacology was taught by seven faculty members in the School of Pharmacy. These included Professor Homer C. Washburn, 1905–11; Professor Charles H. Stocking, 1912–13; Assistant Professor Howard S. Browne, 1913–18; and Professor David B. R. Johnson, 1919–23. In 1924 the subject of pharmacology became a function of the new Department of Biochemistry and Pharmacology, with Mark R. Everett as head for the period 1924–35. In 1935 a separate Department of Pharmacology was formed.

The Department of Preventive Medicine. This department began as a joint Department of Bacteriology and Hygiene in 1912–18, with Gayfree Ellison, M.D., as the head. The name was changed to hygiene and preventive medicine in 1919. Dr. Ellison continued as head from 1919 to 1928. The next change in the department name was to epidemiology and public health in 1929–32, with Dr. Ellison remaining head. Two further changes in the title occurred later, in 1936 to hygiene and public health and in 1944 to preventive medicine and public health.

The Department of Psychiatry and Neurology. The first department of this nature was nervous and mental disorders, headed by Antonio D. Young, M.D., from 1912 to 1915. It was a subsection of the Department of Medicine prior to 1916, at which time it was listed as a separate Department of Mental Diseases and Medical Jurisprudence. John W. Duke, M.D., was head of this department until 1919. In 1920, David Wilson Griffin, M.D., became head of the department. He retained this title until 1940. Neurology was taught as a separate subject by Dr. Young from 1916 to 1930. Dr. James Jackson Gable became acting head of the department for a short period in 1930, and then Dr. Casriel J. Fishman was head of the Department of Neurology from 1930 to 1946. In 1946, the joint Department of Psychiatry and Neurology was formed.

The Department of Radiology. In 1911–12, Everett Samuel Lain, M.D., was professor of dermatology, electrotherapy, and radiography. He was the head of the subdivision of the Department of Surgery labeled radiography. From 1913 to 1915, Dr. Lain continued as head of the Department of Dermatology, Electrotherapy, and Radiography, until 1921 when the department's name was changed to dermatology, electrotherapy, and radiology, and again in 1929 when the name was changed to dermatology and radiology. Two further changes in name occurred, in 1935 the name became dermatology, radiology, and roentgenology, and in 1936 when dermatology and radiology were separated. Dr. Lain served as head of these variously named departments until 1936, at which time John Evans Heatley, M.D., became the head of the new Department of Radiology.

The Department of Urology. From 1911 to 1912 there was a section under medicine named genitourinary, skin, and venereal diseases, with Dr. Curtis R. Day as head until 1913. From 1913 to 1919, Dr. John W. Riley became head of a separate Department of Genitourinary, Skin, and Venereal Diseases. The departmental title was changed in 1916 to genitourinary diseases and syphilology as a separate department. William Jones Wallace, M.D., was head of this department from 1919 to 1934. In 1929 the department title became urology and syphilology, and in 1936, simply urology.

Directors of the Outpatient Staff. Curt Otto Von Wedel, Jr., M.D.,

1911–12; John Smith Hartford, M.D., 1912–14;[1] Cyril Ebert Clymer, M.D., 1917–24; Raymond Lester Murdoch, M.D., 1925–31; and Wann Langston, M.D., 1931–33.

Directors of the School of Nursing. This title was Superintendent of Nursing until 1927. Annette Bourbon Cowles, R.N., 1911–15; Rennette B. Hill, R.N., 1915–16; Edna Holland, G.N., 1916–19; Candice Monfort, G.N., 1919–24; Ada Reitz Crocker, G.N., 1924–27; Mabel E. Smith, M.A., 1928–29; and Candice Monfort Lee, G.N., 1929–37.

Superintendents of the University Hospitals. Annette Bourbon Cowles, R. N., 1911–15; Rennette B. Hill, R.N., 1915–16; H. Mary Workman, R.N., 1916; Paul H. Fesler, acting superintendent, 1916–18, superintendent, 1918–20, fiscal superintendent, 1920–27; Wann Langston, M.D., medical superintendent, 1920–27, superintendent, 1927–31; Henry Hubert Turner, M.D., acting medical superintendent, 1924–25; and John Bodle Smith, M.D., superintendent, 1931–33.

---

[1] As I was unable to determine the director of the outpatient staff for the period 1915–16, I discussed the matter with Dr. John S. Hartford's son, Walter Kenneth Hartford, M.D., at present associate clinical professor of gynecology and obstetrics. He suggested that it was very likely that his father continued to act as director of the outpatient staff until 1916, since that was the year in which he became head of a new separate Department of Gynecology. This very acceptable explanation is supported by the fact that Dr. Hartford made a report for the outpatient department at a September 27, 1915, faculty meeting.

APPENDIX II   Physicians Serving on More Than One Faculty

	Oklahoma City Medical College (1902)	Epworth College of Medicine (1904–10)	Oklahoma Medical College (1907–1909)	Southwest Post-graduate Medical College (1911–15)	University of Oklahoma School of Medicine (1900–)
Andrews, L. E.				X	X
Bevan, W. R.		X		X	
Blesh, A. L.		X		X	X
Bolend, F. J.			X		X
Buxton, L. H.		X		X	X
Dicken, W. E.	X	X		X	
Dixon, W. E.				X	X
Duke, J. W.	X		X	X	X
Edwards, R. T.	X	X		X	X
Ellison, G.			X		
Finney, J. M.		X		X	X
Fullington, W. A.		X	X		
Kuhn, J. F.				X	X
Lain, E. S.		X	X	X	X

	Oklahoma City Medical College (1902)	Epworth College of Medicine (1904–10)	Oklahoma Medical College (1907–1909)	Southwest Post-graduate Medical College (1911–15)	University of Oklahoma School of Medicine (1900–)
Lee, C. E.		X		X	X
Martin, J. T.		X		X	X
Reck, J. A.	X	X			X
Roland, M. M.	X			X	X
Rolater, J. B.	X	X			X
Salmon, W. T.	X	X	X		
Taylor, W. M.			X		X
Todd, H. C.		X		X	X
Walker, D.	X		X		
Wall, G. A.	X		X	X	
Wallace, W. M.		X		X	X
Weir, M. W.		X		X	
West, A. K.	X	X			X
Westfall, L. M.				X	X
White, A. W.		X		X	X
Will, A. A.		X		X	X
Williams, C. W.	X	X			

Executive Order of Governor
William H. Murray, July 27, 1931[1]

WHEREAS, there exists in Oklahoma City a State Institution known as the University Hospital, which hospital is for the treatment of diseases and to supply remedies for sick and suffering citizens of the state and to aid such sick and suffering as by law may be consigned to said hospital by any means or methods that will relieve their suffering, and

WHEREAS, Mrs. W. O. Burgett was placed in said hospital Saturday morning, July 25th, and,

WHEREAS, the medical physicians state that there is very little hope for her recovery, and

WHEREAS, Dr. LeRoy Long has stated to the Governor over the telephone that there is very little hope for her recovery, and

WHEREAS, the husband of said Mrs. Burgett, through the advice of her neighbor and friend, who is a practitioner known as chiropractic, informs him that Mrs. Burgett needs a combined treatment of medicine and chiropractic methods, and

WHEREAS, it is essential that every method be used that would relieve suffering humanity and particularly this patient lodged in a state institution, and

WHEREAS, the said institution is a public institution and should admit all physicians, surgeons and other persons having remedies recognized and licensed by law of the State of Oklahoma, and the denial of the right of the patient and her family to have such treatment is a discrimination in the law between regularly licensed and lawfully permitted attendance upon the sick,

NOW, THEREFORE, I, Wm. H. Murray, Governor of the State of Oklahoma, do hereby direct that the said hospital shall permit any chiropractitioner to treat the said Mrs. Burgett and that the said author-

[1] This is a reproduction of a copy of the original executive order found in the files of the office of the dean.

ities of said institution may be authorized to be present while such treatment is progressing to the end that they may know at all times the condition of the patient. This order is effective at once.

Done this the 27th day of July, 1931
By the Governor of the State of Oklahoma, Wm. H. Murray

ATTEST: R. A. Sneed, Secretary of State
Ina Lee Roberts, Ass't Secretary of State

APPENDIX IV The Faculty of the School of
Medicine, 1910[1]

Norman

Bobo, Charles Sharp, M.D., *dean of the School of Medicine and professor of forensic medicine and therapeutics*

Capshaw, Walter Leander, M.D., *professor of anatomy*

DeBarr, Edwin C., Ph.D., *professor of chemistry*

Hirshfield, Albert Clifford, M.D., *professor of physiology*

Lane, Henry Higgins, M.A., *professor of zoology and embryology*

Maclaren, John Dice, M.D., *professor of physiology and experimental medicine*[2]

Turley, Louis Alvin, M.A., *professor of pathology and neurology*

Washburn, Homer Charles, Ph.C., B.S., *professor of pharmacy and materia medica*

Williams, Guy Yandell, M.A., *associate professor of chemistry*

Oklahoma City (appointed April 13, 1910)

Andrews, Leila Edna, M.D., *instructor in pediatrics*

Bevan, William Richard, M.D., *instructor in therapeutics*

Bisbee, Walter Griswold, M.D., *instructor in orthopedic surgery*

Blesh, Abraham Lincoln, M.D., *professor of surgery and clinical surgery*

Burns, Thomas Craig, M.D., *instructor in nervous and mental diseases*

Buxton, Lauren Haynes, M.D., LL.D., professor of ophthalmology

Cunningham, Samuel Robert, M.D., *professor of gynecology*

1 Following the merger of the Epworth College of Medicine with the university. See *Bulletin of the University of Oklahoma*, New Series, No. 34 (June, 1910), *General Catalog*; the similar *Quarterly Bulletin* in March, 1911; and Gittinger, *The University of Oklahoma*, Appendix III, 201–202. In the 1910 bulletin the private office addresses of the clinical faculty members are given. Since varying, sometimes erroneous, statements are found in letters and compilations concerning this faculty, the author has taken the utmost care in tracing the original official records.

2 Resigned effective January 1, 1911.

Day, Curtis Richard, M.D., *professor of genitourinary and venereal diseases*

Ellison, Gayfree, M.D., *instructor in surgical anatomy*

Ferguson, Edmund Sheppard, M.D., *professor of clinical ophthalmology, otology, rhinology, and laryngology*

Foster, Richard Leland, M.D., *instructor in hygiene, sanitary science, and state medicine*

Hartford, John Smith, M.D., *instructor in gynecology*

Howard, Robert Mayburn, M.D., *professor of clinical surgery*

Jolly, William James, M.D., *professor of principles and practice of surgery*

Lain, Everett Samuel, M.D., *professor of dermatology, electrotherapy, and radiography*

LaMotte, George Althouse, M.D., *professor of clinical medicine*

Lee, Clarence Edward, M.D., *instructor in clinical microscopy*

Looney, Robert Elmore, M.D., *professor of obstetrics*

Martin, Joseph Thomas, M.D., *instructor in obstetrics*

Messenbaugh, Joseph Fife, M.D., *instructor in medicine*

Moorman, Lewis Jefferson, M.D., *professor of physical diagnosis*

Reed, Horace, M.D., *professor of surgical pathology and diagnosis*

Riely, Lea Armistead, M.D., *professor of clinical medicine*

Riley, John William, M.D., *professor of fractures, dislocations, and minor surgery*

Smith, Millington, M.D., *professor of surgery and clinical surgery*

Todd, Harry Coulter, M.D., *professor of otology, rhinology, and laryngology*

West, Archa Kelly, M.D., *professor of principles and practice of medicine*

White, Arthur Weaver, M.D., *instructor in gastrointestinal diseases*

Will, Arthur Anderson, M.D., *instructor in rectal surgery*

Young, Antonio DeBord, M.D., *professor of nervous and mental diseases*

Faculty of the University of Oklahoma
School of Medicine and School of
Nursing Whose Appointments
Terminated Prior to 1932[1]

Allgood, J. M., *assistant in anatomy*, 1925–26

Ambrister, Joseph Campbell, M.D., *instructor in genitourinary, skin, and venereal diseases*, 1911–12

Andreskowski, Wencelaus T., M.D., *assistant in pathology*, 1919

Andrews, Leila Edna, M.D., *assistant professor of pediatrics*, 1910–15

Bailey, William Hotchkiss, M.D., *instructor in clinical pathology*, 1924–25[2]

Bayles, Esther Grace, *dietitian and instructor in dietetics*, 1920–23

Bevan, William Richard, M.D., *assistant professor of obstetrics*, 1910–14

Bisbee, Walter Griswold, M.D., *instructor in orthopedic surgery*, 1910–12

Bobo, Charles Sharp, M.D., *dean of the School of Medicine and professor of forensic medicine and therapeutics*, 1906–11

Bowden, David Thomas, M.D., *assistant professor of epidemiology and public health*, 1929–31

Boyd, Thomas Madison, M.D., *instructor in bacteriology*, 1917[3]

Brewer, Edith, G. N., *instructor in obstetrical nursing*, 1926–27

Browne, Howard Storm, B.A., M.S., *dean of the School of Pharmacy*, 1912–18

Bryant, Homer Lafayette, M.A., *assistant professor of physiology*, 1924–25

Buice, William Alfred, B.S., *assistant professor of bacteriology*, 1926–29

Burnet, Caroline T., G.N., *instructor in practical nursing*, 1928–29

[1] The titles given are those held during the terminating year.
[2] Returned in 1936.
[3] Date determined from military record.

290

Burns, Thomas Craig, M.D., *assistant professor of neurology*, 1910–19

Buxton, Lauren Haynes, M.D., *professor emeritus of otology, rhinology, and laryngology*, 1910–24[4]

Campbell, James Franklin, M.D., *instructor in anatomy*, 1929–30

Capshaw, Walter Leander, M.D., *professor of anatomy*, 1908–15[5]

Chase, Ralph Edward, B.A., B.S., *assistant in physiology*, 1926–28[6]

Cooley, Ben Hunter, M.D., *instructor in minor surgery*, 1922–29

Cottle, Isaac Newton, M.D., *instructor in gynecology*, 1912–13

Cowles, Annette Bourbon, R.N., *superintendent of University Hospital, with rank of instructor*, 1911–15

Crocker, Ada Reitz, G.N., *associate professor of nursing education and director of the School of Nursing*, 1924–27

Darling, John Chester, M.D., *physical director*, 1908–13

Davis, Edward Francis, M.D., *associate professor of ophthalmology*, 1911–28

Day, Curtis Richard, M.D., *dean of the School of Medicine and professor of pathology, serology, and clinical microscopy*, 1910–15

Day, John Lewis, M.D., *instructor in physical diagnosis and minor surgery*, 1920–29

DeBarr, Edwin C., Ph.D., *vice president of the University of Oklahoma and professor of chemistry*, 1900–23

Dickens, Karl La Von, M.S., *instructor in anatomy*, 1929–31

Dickson, Green Knowlton, M.D., *instructor in surgery*, 1925–30

Dixon, Winfield Eugene, M.D., *professor of otology, rhinology, and laryngology*, 1915–30

Duke, John Williams, M.D., *professor of mental diseases and medical jurisprudence*, 1915–20[7]

Else, Frank Lester, B.S., *assistant professor of physiology*, 1929–30

Essenburg, Jacob Martin, Ph.D., *associate professor of anatomy*, 1923–29

Ferguson, Charles Duncan, M.D., *assistant professor of ophthalmology*, 1912–16

Field, Clarence Henry, M.D., *instructor in gynecology*, 1912–13

Finney, Joseph Melville, M.D., *assistant in osteology*, 1905–1906

Fitzgerald, Margaret, G.N., *instructor in surgical technique*, 1929

---

4 Appointment terminated by death.
5 Appointment terminated by death.
6 Returned in 1933.
7 Appointment terminated by death.

Follansbee, Bernice, G.N., *instructor in pediatric nursing*, 1925–26

Foster, Richard Leland, M.D., *assistant professor of medicine*, 1910–14

Foster, Verna, G.N., *instructor in theoretical nursing*, 1928–29

Fowler, William Alonzo, M.D., *professor of obstetrics*, 1912–29

Gastineau, Felix, M.D., *instructor in pathology and clinical microscopy*, 1918–19

Gaston, John Zell, B.S., *assistant professor of anatomy*, 1920–22

Goff, Catherine, *dietitian*, 1919–20

Graham, Stephen Harry, M.D., *assistant in anatomy*, 1915–16

Hall, David Connolly, M.S., *instructor in pharmacology*, 1903–1908

Hamby, Wallace Bernard, B.S., *assistant in histology*, 1924–26

Hamner, Charles Earnest, M.D., *assistant professor of bacteriology*, 1913–14

Hargrove, Reuben Morgan, M.D., *professor of anatomy*, 1916–19

Hartford, John Smith, M.D., *professor of gynecology*, 1910–24[8]

Hawkins, Ada, G.N., *instructor in practical nursing*, 1925–28[9]

Hill, Rennette B., R.N., *superintendent of University Hospital*, 1915–16

Hinnenkamp, Wilhelmina, G.N., *instructor in operating room technique*, 1929–31

Hirshfield, Albert Clifford, M.D., *professor of obstetrics*, 1910–26

Holland, Edna, G.N., *superintendent of University Hospital*, 1916–19

Hoppock, Ruth Evelyn, B.A., *instructor in elementary dietetics*, 1928–30.

Howard, Merle Quest, M.D., *instructor in neurology*, 1923

Hull, Robert Lord, M.D., *associate professor of orthopedic surgery*, 1911–19[10]

Hunter, George, M.D., *instructor in genitourinary diseases and syphilology*, 1914–26

Jansky, Cyril Methodius, B.S., *professor of physics and electrical engineering*, 1905–1908

Jenkins, Joseph Basil, D.D.S., *instructor in dental surgery*, 1923–29

Johnson, David Byars Ray, M.A., *dean of the School of Pharmacy and professor of pharmacy*, 1919–26

[8] Appointment terminated by death.

[9] Returned in 1932.

[10] Appointment terminated by death.

Jolly, William James, M.D., *acting dean of the School of Medicine and professor of surgery*, 1910–14

Knowles, Frank Elwood, Ph.B., *instructor in physics*, 1904–1905

Lane, Henry Higgins, M.A., Ph.D., *professor of zoology and embryology*, 1906–18

Lee, Clarence Edward, M.D., *instructor in clinical microscopy*, 1910–11

Lemmon, William Gladstone, B.S., *assistant in pathology and bacteriology*, 1906–1908

Lewis, Arthur Rimmer, M.D., *special lecturer on applied therapeutics*, 1918–20

Long, LeRoy, M.D., *dean of the School of Medicine and professor of surgery*, 1915–31

Long, LeRoy Downing, M.D., *assistant professor of surgery*, 1924–31[11]

Long, Wendell McLean, M.D., *instructor in gynecology*, 1929–31

Looney, Robert Elmore, M.D., *associate professor of obstetrics*, 1910–29[12]

Mabry, Elba Kenneth, D.D.S., *dentist in outpatient department and instructor in dental surgery*, 1920–21

McDonald, Georgia Helen, *dietitian*, 1919

McGoldrick, Elizabeth, M.A., *instructor in psychiatric social work*, 1930–31

McHenry, Dolph D., M.D., *instructor in otorhinolaryngology and ophthalmology*, 1912–13

Mackenzie, Mary Ard, *superintendent of nurses*, 1919

Maclaren, John Dice, M.D., *professor of physiology and experimental medicine*, 1908–11

McLean, George Davidson, M.D., *instructor in surgery*, 1916–20

Martin, Julia, G.N., *instructor in theoretical nursing*, 1929–30

Mayfield, Warren Troutman, M.D., *instructor in physical diagnosis*, 1926–29

Messenbaugh, Joseph Fife, M.D., *assistant professor of medicine*, 1910–24

Monfort, Candice (Mrs. Candice Monfort Lee), G.N., *superintendent of nurses*, 1919–24, 1929–37

Mueller, Floriene Ann, G.N., *instructor in pediatric nursing*, 1929–30

[11] Returned in 1936.
[12] Appointment terminated by death.

Neill, Alma Jessie, Ph.D., *associate professor of physiology*, 1920–28

Nice, Leonard Blain, Ph.D., *professor of physiology*, 1913–27

Poindexter, Ruth, G.N., *instructor in nursing*, 1924–28

Porter, Earle Sellers, M.A., *instructor in chemistry*, 1912–13

Puckett, Carl, M.D., *special lecturer in public health and sanitation*, 1925–27

Reck, John Arthur, M.D., *assistant professor of gynecology*, 1914–30

Rice, Edgar Elmer, M.D., *assistant professor of gynecology*, 1911–15

Riley, John William, M.D., *professor of genitourinary surgery*, 1910–19

Riley, Robert Hickman, *assistant in pathology and bacteriology*, 1908–1909

Rock, John Lestrange, *laboratory assistant in physiology*, 1912–13

Rolater, Joseph Brown, M.D., *lecturer in clinical surgery*, 1911–12

Rue, John Davison, Jr., M.A., *associate professor of chemistry*, 1911–13

Russell, Glen Alexander, M.D., *instructor in anatomy*, 1930–31

Sapper, Herbert Victor Louis, B.S., B.A., *instructor in bacteriology*, 1912–15

Seymour, James, Ph.C., *instructor in pharmacy*, 1904

Slatkin, Harry, *laboratory assistant in anatomy*, 1912–13

Smith, Mabel E., M.A., *associate professor of nursing education and director of the School of Nursing*, 1928–29

Smith, Ralph Vernon, M.D., *assistant professor of surgery*, 1911–15

Smith, Wendal Doop, M.S., *assistant professor of histology and embryology*, 1926–28

Sorgatz, Frank Bruner, M.D., *associate professor of clinical pathology and research*, 1911–18[13]

Soutar, Richard Gray, B.A., B.S., *professor of physical education*, 1914–17

Steele, Julia Elizabeth (Mrs. Julia Steele Eley), B.A., B.S., *instructor in pathology*, 1919–25

Stephenson, Joseph Clark, Ph.D., M.D., *professor of anatomy*, 1919–31

Stocking, Charles Howard, Ph.D., *dean of the School of Pharmacy and professor of pharmacy*, 1912–13

[13] Appointment terminated by death.

Stone, Merlin Jones, M.D., *associate professor of anatomy*, 1920–23
Stoops, Roy Philson, M.D., *acting dean of the School of Medicine and professor of anatomy.* 1903–1908
Stout, Marvin Elroy, M.D., *instructor in surgery*, 1916–21
Taylor, Pleasant Addison, *laboratory assistant in anatomy and physiology*, 1911–13
Torrey, John Paine, M.D., *acting professor of anatomy*, 1915–20
Townsend, Myron Thomas, Ph.D., *associate professor of histology and embryology*, 1928–30
Upjohn, Lawrence Northcote, M.D., *head of the School of Medicine and professor of anatomy and pathology*, 1900–1904
Van Vleet, Albert Heald, Ph.D., *professor of biology and dean of the Graduate School*, 1900–1909
Von Wedel, Curt Otto, Jr., M.D., *assistant professor of surgery*, 1912–16
Warner, Francis James, M.D., *associate professor of anatomy*, 1924–25
Washburn, Homer Charles, B.S., Ph.C., *dean of the School of Pharmacy and professor of pharmacy and materia medica*, 1904–11
Watson, Leigh Festus, M.D., *assistant professor of surgery*, 1911–17
Weber, Flora, G.N., *instructor in nursing education and assistant director of the School of Nursing*, 1925–29
West, Archa Kelly, M.D., *professor of medicine*, 1910–25[14]
Wickham, Mallalieu McCullagh, M.A., *instructor in histology and pathology*, 1922–24
Wilber, Gertrude Helen, M.D., *assistant professor of histology and embryology*, 1930–31
Will, Arthur Anderson, M.D., *associate professor of rectal surgery*, 1910–26[15]
Williams, Edward Marsh, B.S., *instructor in pathology and bacteriology*, 1905–1908
Williams, Guy Yandell, M.S., *associate professor of chemistry*, 1906–12
Williams, Robert Findlater, M.D., *dean of the School of Medicine and professor of clinical medicine*, 1911–13
Workman, Mary H., R.N., *superintendent of University Hospital*, 1916
Yeakel, Earl LeRoy, *instructor in bacteriology*, 1917–18

[14] Appointment terminated by death.
[15] Appointment terminated by death.

Young, Andrews Marriman, M.D., *instructor in obstetrics*, 1912–17
Young, Antonio DeBord, M.D., *professor of neurology*, 1910–30[16]
Zimmerman, Martha Eggleston, R.N., *assistant superintendent of University Hospital, with rank of instructor*, 1912–14

[16] Appointment terminated by death.

Index

302

The paper on which this book is printed bears the watermark of the University of Oklahoma Press and has an effective life of at least three hundred years.